CHECK CD-ROM IN BACK POCKET

Clinics in Developmental Medicine No. 159
GROSS MOTOR FUNCTION MEASURE
(GMFM-66 AND GMFM-88)
USER'S MANUAL

© 2002 Mac Keith Press

High Holborn House, 52–54 High Holborn, London WC1V 6RL

Senior Editor: Martin C.O. Bax
Editor: Hilary M. Hart
Managing Editor: Michael Pountney
Sub Editor: Pat Chappelle

First published in this edition 2002

British Library Cataloguing-in-Publication data:
A catalogue record for this book is available from the British Library

ISSN: 0069 4835
ISBN: 1 89868329 8

Printed by The Lavenham Press Ltd, Water Street, Lavenham, Suffolk
Mac Keith Press is supported by Scope

Clinics in Developmental Medicine No. 159

Gross Motor Function Measure (GMFM-66 & GMFM-88) User's Manual

DIANNE J RUSSELL
PETER L ROSENBAUM
LISA M AVERY
MARY LANE

CanChild Centre for Childhood Disability Research
McMaster University
Hamilton, Ontario
Canada

2002
Mac Keith Press

Distributed by 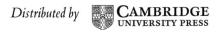 CAMBRIDGE
UNIVERSITY PRESS

AUTHORS' APPOINTMENTS

Dianne J Russell   Associate Professor, School of Rehabilitation Science, Faculty of Health Sciences, McMaster University; *and* Research Co-ordinator, *CanChild* Centre for Childhood Disability Research, Hamilton, Ontario, Canada

Peter L Rosenbaum   Professor of Paediatrics, Faculty of Health Sciences, McMaster University; Co-Director, *CanChild* Centre for Childhood Disability Research; Canada Research Chair in Child-hood Disability, Hamilton, Ontario, Canada

Lisa M Avery   Master of Science (Statistics) Candidate, University of Ontago, Dunedin, New Zealand; *and* Research Assistant, *CanChild* Centre for Childhood Disability Research, Hamilton, Ontario, Canada

Mary Lane   Pediatric Physiotherapist and Clinical Consultant, *CanChild* Centre for Childhood Disability Research, Hamilton, Ontario, Canada

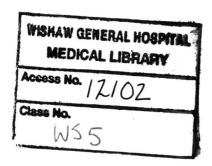

CONTENTS

ACKNOWLEDGEMENTS

The current GMFM manual is in fact the third (and we hope much improved) version of work that has been ongoing since the late 1980s. The original manual was prepared in 1990 and a second edition appeared in 1993. In both versions we acknowledged people whose efforts had contributed to the work. These included, of course, the authors of the original publication describing the GMFM (Carolyn Gowland, Susan Hardy, Nancy Plews, Heather McGavin, David Cadman and Sheila Jarvis). We wish to thank Kate O'Connor Steel who shared with us her Motor Control Assessment where many of the items for the GMFM originated. In addition we recognized clinical colleagues and a number of students and support staff who had participated in the creation of the work then available. They number too many to cite individually, but we are very grateful that they supported our early efforts to create a new clinical assessment tool.

A number of McMaster University faculty colleagues provided signal input into the early conception of the GMFM through either conceptual or technical support. They include Drs Charlie Goldsmith, Gordon Guyatt, David Streiner and Christal Woodward, all acknowledged experts in clinical epidemiology and measurement development. Each gave freely of their time and ideas as the GMFM took shape in the mid-1980s. The recent Rasch analysis work would not have been possible without the statistical and methodological expertise of Drs Stephen Walter and Parminder Raina, who spent many meetings poring over Rasch outputs and discussing issues as we worked our way through this relatively new approach to measurement. Dr Bob Palisano provided invaluable advice and feedback on many aspects of this work, as did Dr Steve Hanna.

A project to create and validate a clinical measure requires the efforts of literally dozens of dedicated clinical colleagues who toil in the trenches to collect the raw data that are shaped by the research team. These people—mainly clinical physiotherapists in the Children's Treatment Centres associated with the Ontario Association of Children's Rehabilitation Services (OACRS)—have participated in the Ontario Motor Growth Curve study since 1996. Between them they have done over 3000 GMFMs that provided the basic materials for the work reported here. They participated in the GMFM training program and tolerated repeated reassessments of their reliability with patience and enthusiasm. We are forever in their debt, because this work could clearly not have been done without them. We also recognize that clinical research is an 'add-on' for many OACRS centres, and thank the Executive Directors for their partnership in research ventures like this one.

CanChild Centre for Childhood Disability Research has been supported since 1989 by the Health System-Linked Research Units program of the Research Branch of the Ontario Ministry of Health and Long-Term Care. Work such as that reported here would be difficult if not impossible without the continuing support of this program, for which we are most grateful. The research data collection activities of the therapists were made possible through the generous grant support of both the Medical Research Council of Canada (now the

Canadian Institutes of Health Research) and the National Center for Medical Rehabilitation Research of the National Institute of Child Health and Human Development at NIH (grant R01-HD-34947). Barbara Galuppi coordinated all aspects of this multi-site five-year study with admirable skill and efficiency, and in this way has made an enormous contribution to all the work of our research group. Of course were it not for the unique contribution of time and effort of hundreds of children with cerebral palsy and their families, completing questionnaires and permitting videotaping of their activities, this work would have been impossible.

Colleagues from around the world have participated in GMFM training workshops and helped us in our work through a combination of perceptive suggestions, insightful questions, the use of the GMFM in their clinical and research efforts, and generous sharing of their experiences and often their data. At the risk of missing some people, we wish to recognize in particular Kristie Bjornson at Children's Hospital and Regional Medical Centre, Seattle, and Marjolijn Ketelaar at Utrecht University. Drs Suzann Campbell at the University of Illinois at Chicago and Steve Haley of Boston University were very helpful in the early phases of our project, sharing perspectives from their Rasch analysis experiences with the TIMP and the PEDI, respectively. The work reported here thus has a truly international flavour, and we appreciate the support of these friends.

Having created a Gross Motor Ability Estimator (GMAE) computer program to score the GMFM-66, we wished to assess whether the program could be applied and interpreted by clinical therapists outside of a research environment. We are indebted to the many therapists in OACRS programs who helped to pilot test the several versions of the program as we worked to make it accessible. Dr Doreen Bartlett, Lisa Rivard, Marilyn Wright and Virginia Wright were particularly helpful in offering insightful feedback which we have used to improve the program.

Thanks to Eric Bosch and Graham Passmore for their programming expertise in turning our GMFM training videotapes into the interactive GMFM CD-ROM teaching tool that is now available for self-training in the use of the GMFM.

We wish finally to acknowledge the encouragement and help we receive every day from our colleagues at *CanChild*, who have tolerated our apparently endless efforts to complete this work, perhaps to the neglect of other responsibilities! Particular thanks go to Betsy Spencer, Pat Abernathy and Kamal Mangat who have been unofficial members of the Motor Measures Group, and whose behind-the-scenes contributions we know better than most people.

The unsung heroes of an effort like this are our families, who patiently accepted our unavailability as we pored over endless drafts, revisions and proofs of this book. We wish to recognize and thank them for indulging our passion for measurement and for allowing us the luxury of using our energies to see this work through to completion.

At the end of the day, of course, with all the help and support we have received from people named and unnamed, any shortcomings in this work are the responsibility of the authors.

2
CONCEPTUAL BACKGROUND

Cerebral palsy

Cerebral palsy (CP) refers to a group of non-progressive disorders of the development of motor control occurring as a result of damage to the developing central nervous system before, during or relatively soon after the time of birth (Mutch *et al*. 1992). CP has highly variable effects on the neurological and functional development of the child, effects that impact on the degree of impairment, activity limitations and participation. In its recent revisions of the 1980 International Classification of Impairments, Disabilities and Handicaps, the World Health Organization describes activities as "the nature and extent of functioning at the level of the person" (WHO 2001). Activity limitations (formerly referred to as "disabilities") are those restrictions or lack of ability to perform an activity in a manner or within the range that is considered normal for that age and stage of development (WHO 2001). The principal activity limitations resulting from CP involve problems in motor function, with associated problems often occurring in the cognitive, social and communicative domains (Kennes *et al*. 2002). Gross and fine motor function measures provide quantification of the degree of physical disability.

Measuring gross motor function

The measurement of gross motor function in children with CP, as in other neurodevelopmental disorders in children, is a complex process. Although the child with CP will mature motorically to a greater or lesser extent, motor development and the acquisition of motor skills are almost always delayed or disordered. Motor development may plateau for short or long periods of time, movements may become atypical, and in unfavourable circumstances, regression in motor milestones may occur. Typical gross motor developmental milestones are well documented in the literature and these form the basis of the items in the five dimensions in the Gross Motor Function Measure. The items include lying activities in prone and supine, progressing to rolling, sitting, kneeling, crawling and standing, and ultimately walking, running and jumping. Within each dimension, activities reflective of the special problems of children with CP have been selected.

Numerous treatment approaches have been promoted to address the motor function difficulties of children with CP. With a few exceptions, however, the value of these techniques has yet to be clearly established with methodologically sound research. One of the many challenges in assessing the effectiveness of therapies has been the paucity of validated measures of function that have been shown to be responsive to important change in the functions of interest. In a review of measures used in published controlled clinical trials of physical therapy interventions for children with CP, Rosenbaum *et al*. (1990) highlighted the limitations of measures available at that time. Since then several measures of motor function have been developed and validated for assessing infants. These include the Test of Infant Motor Performance (TIMP) (Campbell *et al.* 1993), the Alberta Infant Motor Scale (AIMS) (Piper and Darrah 1994) and the revised Bayley Scales of Infant Development (BSID-II) (Bayley 1993). New measures for children with developmental disabilities include the Pediatric Evaluation of Disability Inventory (PEDI) (Haley *et al.* 1992) and the Motor Control Assessment (Steel *et al.* 1991). Other tools that have broadened the perspective from traditional functional activities to encompass the level of participation include the School Function Assessment (Coster *et al.* 1998), the Child Health Questionnaire (Landgraf *et al.* 1996) and the Activity Scale for Kids (Young *et al.* 2000). As a help to users of childhood disability measures, a CD-ROM program has been developed that uses the modified ICIDH framework to help clinicians understand, evaluate and choose appropriate pediatric outcome measures from a database of over 125 measures that have been critically reviewed for their clinical usefulness and psychometric properties (Law *et al.* 1999).

GENERAL ISSUES IN MEASUREMENT
Construction and validation of a measure must be predicated upon its ultimate purpose. Methodological rigor is essential from the conception of the measure to the completion of its development and testing.

PURPOSES OF MEASURES
Guyatt *et al.* (1992) have provided a methodological framework for assessing health measures. They point out that measures may be used for one or more purposes. A *discriminative* measure distinguishes between individuals with and without a particular characteristic or function. For example, the Peabody Developmental Motor Scales (Folio *et al.* 1983) are used to categorize children into centile rank scores, standard scores or age-equivalent scores. A *predictive* measure provides an estimate of prognosis or future status. Thus the Bleck scale (Bleck 1975) predicts ambulation at age 7 years on the basis of a preschool child's postural and tonic reflex activity at around age 2 years. An *evaluative* measure is needed to measure the magnitude of change in function over time or after treatment, as was attempted with the measure used by Wright and Nicholson (1973) to assess several motor-related clinical functions before and after a period of physical therapy.

Measures generally are developed and validated specifically to fulfil one of the functions described above. A measure should not automatically be used for a purpose other than the one for which it was created, or applied to a population dissimilar to the one on which it was developed and validated. For example, Bleck's predictive measure (Bleck 1975) will not suffice as a discriminative instrument. Bleck's explicit purpose was to develop a test to predict future ambulation based on the presence or absence of seven postural and reflex items, and the scale has excellent measurement properties to accomplish this task (sensitivity = 0.98; specificity = 0.84). Seven items would not, however, be adequate to distinguish or discriminate a population of children with CP into anything other than very crude categories, because the scope and subtlety of motor behaviour in this population require much finer distinctions than can be achieved with such a small subsample of the domain of motor function. Similarly, as an evaluative measure, the Bleck scale is limited both by the number of items potentially responsive to change in motor function with time and treatment, and by the narrow range of response options (present/absent) by which to annotate improved motor function.

CHARACTERISTICS OF AN EVALUATIVE MEASURE

To assess the effectiveness of treatment on motor function outcomes for children with CP, an evaluative measure with specific structural characteristics is required.

A. Items in the measure must be selected on the basis of both clinical relevance and potential responsiveness to change. For example, a therapist might reasonably anticipate a change in duration of independent standing ability of a 5-year-old following a physical therapy program, but would be quite unlikely to expect a change in the asymmetric tonic neck reflex (ATNR) of the same child. It would be appropriate, therefore, to include duration of standing but not ATNR in an evaluative measure, despite the clinical importance of both to overall motor behaviour. Because change in the ATNR over time is not expected to occur, measuring this item will be unhelpful as a means of detecting change in motor function. Its presence in the evaluative measure serves no purpose and it might even add measurement error to the instrument.

B. The measure must be feasible to use in terms of the time required to administer and score it, patient acceptance and cost. There need to be clearly described standardized instructions, mutually exclusive and collectively exhaustive response options, and explicit scaling.

C. The measure must be reliable; that is, it must give consistent responses or scores when used repeatedly by the same assessor over time, or with different (trained) observers evaluating 'stable' subjects.

D. The measure must be valid; that is, responsive to real change and stable in the absence of change. The essential component in validating an evaluative instrument is to establish its responsiveness to change.

In summary, an evaluative measure must contain relevant items and must be applicable to the population on whom it is to be used, feasible to administer, reliable and valid. An important aspect of the validation of an evaluative measure is evidence of the measure's ability to demonstrate responsiveness to clinically important change over time.

NORM-REFERENCED VS CRITERION-REFERENCED TESTS

Clinical measures are usually either "norm-referenced" or "criterion-referenced". A norm-referenced measure is constructed using data derived from measures taken on a sample of the population on which the instrument is meant to be used. Assumptions of distributional normality are implicit in this type of measure, and the measured characteristics of individuals (for example height or weight) are compared to the "norm" for that population. These comparisons may be expressed as centiles, quartiles or other categorical quantifications. It is possible to create norm-referenced measures for special populations, such as the charts that are available to plot the growth patterns of children with Down syndrome (Cronk *et al.* 1988). Measures designed to discriminate are almost always norm-referenced. Examples of norm-referenced pediatric motor measures include the Peabody Developmental Motor Scales

(Folio *et al.* 1983), the Test of Infant Motor Performance (TIMP) (Campbell *et al.* 1993), the Alberta Infant Motor Scale (AIMS) (Piper and Darrah 1994), and the revised Bayley Scales of Infant Development (BSID-II) (Bayley 1993).

Criterion-referenced measures are developed by choosing items relevant to the domain of interest, and then describing the criterion by which the observer can assess whether that characteristic or functional attribute is present (or perhaps the extent to which it is present, where gradations of the criterion are explicitly described). Note that the frame of reference for comparison here is the presence or absence of the characteristic (or functional activity) of interest, rather than a comparison with the general population. Examples of criterion-referenced assessments that include motor function include the Functional Independence Measure for Children (WeeFim®) (WeeFim 2000), the PEDI (Haley *et al.* 1992) and the Gross Motor Function Measure (Russell *et al.* 1989).

LEVEL OF MEASUREMENT SCALE: ORDINAL OR INTERVAL

Evaluative measures may use either ordinal or interval scoring systems. Streiner and Norman (1989) discuss the differences between these two types of scores and the descriptive statistics that are appropriate for each. An *ordinal* measure presents a number of response options that "order" the characteristic of interest from better to less skilled performance. There is no assumption that the relative distances between adjacent categories on such a scale are equal to one another. The Gross Motor Function Classification System (GMFCS) (Palisano *et al.* 1997) and the Functional Independence Measure for Children (WeeFim®) (WeeFim 2000) provide examples of such a scaling approach. Non-parametric statistics are recommended to summarize ordinal data.

An *interval* scale is one in which the distances between adjacent categories are equal throughout the measure. For example, the measure of a child's height is made using a meter stick. The one centimetre interval is constant along the entire length of the meter stick and is understood universally. Interval scales can be summarized using parametric statistics.

RASCH ANALYSIS: MODIFYING AN ORDINAL MEASURE TO GIVE INTERVAL SCORES

It is possible to achieve interval scores from an ordinal measure. An area of statistics known as *item response theory*, and in particular *Rasch analysis*, is concerned with this goal. Using empirical data Rasch analysis places *items* along an interval continuum of difficulty and *subjects* along an interval continuum of ability.

Placing items along a difficulty continuum reveals the hierarchical structure of the items and allows clinicians more easily to target items that are likely to be within the current functional range of the child. This approach also provides information about the relative difficulty of the items and even the relative difficulty of the steps (response options) within each item, something that is not possible with standard ordinal scaling.

By placing subjects along an interval continuum it is possible to track a child's progress more meaningfully. In an ordinal measure, such as the GMFM-88, using a percentage achieved as the score, an improvement in percent score from 10% to 20% is not necessarily equal to the change from a score of 20% to 30%. In fact, it is very likely that a change of score from 20% to 30% is *less* of an improvement than a change of score from 10% to 20%.

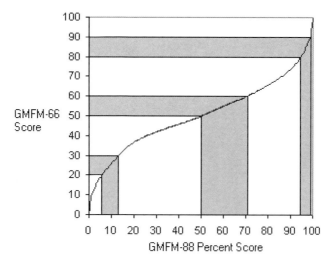

Fig. 2.1. Ogive curve demonstrating how a 10-point change on the interval scale of the GMFM-66 relates to different amounts of change on the GMFM-88 depending on whether one is measuring in the middle or at the ends of the scale.

This is because items tend to be clumped in the middle of the measure with fewer items measuring behaviors at the extremes of the scale. Figure 2.1 is an ogive curve showing the general relationship between ordinal summary scores and interval-level Rasch scores. Note that 10 units of true *interval-level* change (displayed on the ordinate of the graph) correspond to very different amounts of *ordinal-level* change (displayed on the abscissa) at different areas of the measure.

VALIDATION OF AN EVALUATIVE MEASURE
A brief review of the three major types of validity will be presented before discussion of the issues relevant to validation of an evaluative measure.

CONTENT VALIDITY
Content validity is based on whether the items of an instrument adequately represent the domain they are supposed to measure (Kaplan *et al.* 1976). This test domain is known as the underlying *construct* or *latent trait* of the measure. Content validity is usually the first step in developing a measure for further validation. Establishing content validity is not, however, sufficient validation for a measure unless it is based on empirical testing. Classical test theory uses expert opinion to determine if the measure (and individual items) do in fact measure the assumed construct. Conversely, Rasch analysis uses statistical testing, in the form of the goodness-of-fit statistics, to determine how well items measure the latent trait (or the characteristic being measured). If the majority of items in a measure (more than 95%) do measure the latent trait then the measure is said to be *unidimensional*. Unidimensionality is a requirement for a valid interval measure.

7

CRITERION VALIDITY

Criterion validity can be established only when there currently exists a measure (the criterion) that can accurately assess the phenomenon of interest and to which the new measure can be compared. Unfortunately, for discriminative or evaluative indices there is rarely a "criterion" or "gold standard" and this is often the reason for developing a new measure! Abstract variables or concepts have no criterion and must therefore be operationally defined and validated by the method of construct validation.

CONSTRUCT VALIDITY

Construct validation requires the definition of the abstract concept or theory (in the current case, gross motor function) and a choice of indicators (observable and measurable characteristics) to represent that concept. Next one develops *a priori* hypotheses about how the measure should work if it is in fact measuring the construct of interest. Each hypothesis is then tested using data. It must be emphasized that one does not prove a measure is valid; rather one gathers evidence to demonstrate that the indicators chosen actually measure the abstract concept. In this sense, establishing validity is an ongoing process. The more evidence one accumulates by using different methods, the more certain one can be regarding the validity of the measure.

RESPONSIVENESS

Responsiveness is an important part of validating a measure whose intended purpose is to measure change over time. Responsiveness has been identified as the key feature of an evaluative measure in order to determine whether it will be useful in measuring clinically important change over time (Kirshner and Guyatt 1985). Responsiveness is evaluated by determining the ability or power of the test to detect a minimal clinically important change in function.

Recent interest in techniques to measure functional change has led to a number of approaches to establishing responsiveness of evaluative clinical measures (Lipsey 1983, Deyo and Inui 1984, Meenan *et al.* 1984, Deyo and Centor 1986, Guyatt *et al.* 1987). Stratford *et al.* (1996) provide a thorough summary and critique of the various strategies for assessing change over time.

RELIABILITY

Reliability or reproducibility is defined as the degree of consistency or dependability of a measure (Streiner and Norman 1989) and is assessed by correlating at least two sets of scores. Common examples include intra-rater and inter-rater reliability, test–retest, and split-half or alternate forms reliability. The assumption underlying traditional reliability measures (*e.g.* Pearson's r) is that a test score is composed of a true score which represents the actual level of the trait being measured and an error score which is random and independent of the true score (Nunnally 1978). By definition, this assumes that all error is non-systematic or random; however, there may also be systematic error or bias as illustrated in the equation below (Chambers and Haines 1982):

MEASURED VALUE = TRUE VALUE + SYSTEMATIC ERROR + RANDOM ERROR.

Measurement error (both systematic and random) must be decreased as much as possible to get the best indication of the true value. Possible sources of measurement error are numerous and vary with the particular design of a study. These will generally include factors within and between observers, within subjects and within the environment, as well as error in the measurement instrument.

Another way to express reliability is to relate the true score variance to the total variance (true score variance plus error variance). By this definition, the true score variance is as important in determining the size of the reliability coefficient as is the error variance (Mitchell 1979) and the reliability will increase when the sample subjects are more heterogeneous (*i.e.* high true score variance in test scores between individuals). An intra-class correlation coefficient (ICC) based on analysis of variance has been the statistic of choice for reliability using interval (and sometimes ordinal) data because it allows for different variance components to be identified. An ICC may take into account variance from sources other than individual differences and measurement error (*e.g.* occasions, scorers, subjects and the interactions among these factors).

If external criterion measures are being used for validation then another concern is whether the external criterion measures are reliable. For example, if change on the new measure is being compared to change as judged by a parent, it is important to determine whether parents are consistent in their ratings from one time to the next when no "real" change has occurred.

Summary
There are many ways to gather evidence about the reliability and validity of measures. In addition to traditional methods of establishing validity it is also important to evaluate the responsiveness to change of measures whose primary purpose is evaluative. Measures that have interval scaling allow for more precise measurement for both descriptive and evaluative purposes than ordinal scales and satisfy assumptions for many higher level statistical analyses.

3
DEVELOPMENT AND VALIDATION OF THE GMFM-88

Test construction

ITEM SELECTION

Selection of items for the original GMFM was based on a literature review and judgments of clinicians at the participating centres. The published version of the GMFM contains 88 items. Several items were drawn from the Motor Control Assessment (unpublished when work was begun on the GMFM in 1984, subsequently published by Steel *et al.* 1991), and from the work of Hoskins and Squires (1973). Items judged to be measurable, clinically important and with the potential to show change in function in children normally seen at children's treatment centres were included. All items could usually be accomplished by a 5-year-old with typically developing motor abilities. Since treatment goals are generally directed towards maximizing a child's potential to become as independent as possible, it was considered important to determine whether a child could complete the task independently, without any "hands on" assistance from another person. It was also recognized that reliability would likely be better if observations of motor function were made without the direct hands-on involvement of the assessor.

For ease of administration the items were initially grouped on the rating form by test position and arranged in a developmental sequence, based on clinical judgment. For scoring purposes items were aggregated to represent five separate dimensions of motor function. Prone and supine items were combined to represent "Lying & Rolling"; 4-point and kneeling items were combined to represent "Crawling & Kneeling"; "Sitting" and "Standing" items were considered separately; and the walking, running and stair climbing items represented the "Walking, Running & Jumping" dimension.

The original GMFM, used in the field testing and described by Russell *et al.* (1989), had 85 items. After the measure was published, further minor modifications were made. These included adding three items (to ensure that unilateral function was assessed on each side of the body and not just on one, as had been the case with the original 85-item version).

It was also important to assess the reliability of the 88-item version versus the 85-item version. This was done using a balanced incomplete block research design with a sample of 16 therapists who did a total of 64 assessments, half using the 85-item version and half the 88-item version. The reliability values using the GMFM-88 guidelines reached acceptable levels for all dimensions and the total score based on an intra-class correlation coefficient (ICC) greater than 0.75. The results from this small study assured us that the GMFM-88 was comparable to the old version and could be used in its place. The GMFM-88 was available for clinical use from 1990.

ITEM SCORING

Scoring of each GMFM item is done using a consistent generic four-point ordinal scale. Values of 0 to 3 are assigned to the four categories:

      0 = does not initiate (the task being tested)

      1 = initiates (<10% of the task)

      2 = partially completes (10% to <100% of the task)

      3 = completes (the task as outlined in the criterion descriptions).

     NT = not tested.*

    The administration and scoring guidelines contain explicit definitions for partial and complete achievement of each item, and are *essential for proper administration and scoring*. A six page score sheet is used to record results.

Validity of the GMFM-88

CONTENT VALIDITY

Therapists from the Children's Developmental Rehabilitation Programme (CDRP) at Chedoke-McMaster Hospitals in Hamilton, Ontario, and from the Hugh Macmillan Rehabilitation Centre (HMRC) in Toronto, Ontario, were involved in the pilot testing of the GMFM. Therapists from both centres attended a number of group meetings to give feedback regarding the items and the format. A score sheet was designed along with a booklet of guidelines including item definitions and a scoring key. A list of the equipment needed to complete the test was included with directions for administering the GMFM. This version of the GMFM was used for the validation study (Russell *et al.* 1989).

PRE-TESTING OF THERAPISTS

Once the final version of the GMFM was ready, therapists were encouraged to practice with children in their clinical caseload. A videotape was prepared to test therapists to a criterion level of reliability prior to enrolling subjects in the validation study. The criterion tape showed partial GMFM assessments of three children. These children were chosen to represent various levels of function in order to illustrate items from all areas of the GMFM. The therapists had to reach at least 70% raw agreement with a criterion score to be able to commence enrolling children in the study. No credit was given for partial agreement and scores were not corrected for chance. Feedback was given to all therapists on discrepancies between their score and the criterion scoring. Twelve of 13 therapists reached criterion on the first trial.

THE VALIDATION STUDY

A study was designed to validate the GMFM for its capability to detect change in gross motor function. It was not designed to evaluate any specific therapy, and children were expected to continue the treatment they were normally receiving. A standardized GMFM was administered by the same trained therapist twice over several months, and change

---

*The Not Tested category was not in the original GMFM validation but will now be part of the GMFM-88 and GMFM-66 Score Sheet. For the GMFM-88 scoring the NT category will receive a score of 0.

TABLE 3.1
Sample characteristics—numbers of subjects by diagnosis, age and severity

Diagnosis	Age (years)				Total
	<3	3–<6	6–<9	≥9	
Cerebral palsy	32	38	32	9	111
Mild	8	13	6	2	29
Moderate	13	16	13	4	46
Severe	11	9	13	3	36
Acquired brain injury	1	2	5	17	25
Typically developing	30	4	0	0	34

scores were correlated with independent judgments of change in motor function made by parents, therapists and "masked" video observers.

In addition to the sample of children with CP we chose to add two other groups of children to our validation sample. Typically developing young children under 5 years of age, and children who had experienced a recent brain injury, were both groups of children where, in the majority of cases, relatively large changes in motor function could be expected over the six months of the study.

Some of the children with CP were scheduled for surgery during the time of the study and they provided a unique opportunity to see whether the GMFM was responsive to changes in both directions. For example, by assessing a child one extra time (*i.e.* two weeks postoperatively after cast removal, when the expectation would be decreased motor function) both positive and negative change could be evaluated. This case example is included in the validation article (Russell *et al.* 1989).

VALIDATION STUDY SAMPLE
A referral form was completed by the child's regular treating therapist. In addition to age and sex, therapists were asked to describe the type and distribution of CP, to judge its severity (at that time the terms "mild", "moderate" and "severe" were used without explicit definitions), and to estimate the child's cognitive function. Information about therapy included duration, frequency and current goals of the physical therapy programme. Parent information included demographic data on the child and on the family structure.

Subject sample
The total validation sample included children with CP, children with acquired brain injury, and typically developing preschoolers with no known physical disabilities. Table 3.1 shows the sample characteristics by diagnosis, age and severity.

• *Cerebral palsy (CP):* One hundred and eleven children with a diagnosis of CP made by a neurodevelopmental pediatrician were included in the study. The mean age at first GMFM assessment was 4.9 years, varying from 5 months to 15.4 years. The severity of CP (mild/moderate/severe) was judged clinically by the therapist and these three groups were sampled

TABLE 3.2
Classification of sample according to type
of cerebral palsy (CP)

Type	n	%
Spastic CP	88	79.2
Diplegia	38	34.2
Quadriplegia	33	29.7
Hemiplegia	16	14.4
Triplegia	1	0.9
Non-spastic CP	23	20.7
Athetosis	14	12.6
Mixed	6	5.4
Hypotonia	2	1.8
Ataxia	1	0.9

approximately equally. Younger age groups (<3 years and 3–5 years) were intentionally oversampled in order to include a larger proportion of children more likely to change in motor function.

Forty-five per cent of the children with CP had normal intelligence as judged by their treating therapist; 30.6% were classified as slow learners, 16.2% as mildly retarded and 6.3% as moderately to severely retarded; and 1.8% had missing data. The classification of CP according to type is shown in Table 3.2.

• *Acquired Brain Injury (ABI):* Twenty-five individuals recovering in hospital from acute head injury were enrolled (Table 3.1). The mean age at first GMFM assessment was 12.5 years, varying from 2.8 years to 22.8 years. The expectation was that improvement in motor function over the time frame of the study in this group would in the majority of cases be substantial, and thus increase the number of dramatic changes in motor function assessed.

(3) *Typically developing (TD):* Thirty-four children under 5 years of age with no known motor problems were also included in the study. The mean age at first GMFM assessment was 1.3 years, varying from 1 month to 4.3 years. It is important to note that the scores from these children do not constitute a normative sample; rather they were included to provide support for the validation hypotheses. These children (Table 3.1) were a convenience volunteer sample.

Therapist sample
Thirteen therapists, all of whom had reached criterion on the GMFM, participated in the validation study—seven from the Hugh Macmillan Rehabilitation Centre (Toronto, ON) and six from the Children's Developmental Rehabilitation Program (Hamilton, ON). They had a mean of 7.9 years pediatric experience that varied from less than one year to 28 years.

Face validity
Following the validation study, a questionnaire was circulated to all 13 therapists involved

with the study. Results indicated that therapists were satisfied with both the content of the GMFM and the four-point scaling system. Therapists also indicated that the GMFM appeared to be a useful discriminative measure aiding in treatment planning and parent education.

Validation of responsiveness
In the absence of an accepted criterion or gold standard evaluative measure of motor function for the target population, validation of the responsiveness of the GMFM had to be established using a construct validation process. This was done by testing *a priori* hypotheses about how change scores on the GMFM would relate to change scores on other measures that were judged to be assessing the same thing. Three measures were chosen for the comparison: parents' rating of change in gross motor performance; physical therapists' rating of change; and change as assessed by independent therapists viewing videotapes randomized with respect to the before/after status of the children being assessed.

Parent and therapist ratings of change were done using a standardized questionnaire. In order to obtain an independent rating of change from therapists, 28 paired videotapes of children being assessed with the GMFM six months apart were viewed by therapists familiar with the GMFM, but unfamiliar with these children. Therapist observers were "masked" to the order in which the tapes were presented (earlier vs later). After viewing a pair of tapes, the observer completed a standardized questionnaire similar to that used with parents and the child's regular therapists, to judge change.

The *first hypothesis* stated that correlations between change scores on the GMFM and "masked" therapists' judgments of change on videotaped assessments would be greater than 0.45, and greater than correlations with judgments made by treating therapists; correlations with parent judgments would be lowest at 0.30–0.45.

This *a priori* judgment about the magnitude of the correlations was based on discussions with methodologist colleagues who had worked in related areas of measurement design. The rationale was that the video assessment is the most objective assessment and is looking strictly at actual performance ("does do" rather than "can do"); in addition, both the videos were viewed within two hours, so that the independent therapist would have a visual reminder of performance rather than a verbal one. We hypothesized that treating physical therapists' assessments of change were likely to be based upon both what the child *does* achieve and what they *can* achieve according to the therapist's knowledge of the child's potential. Therefore, the physical therapists' assessment of change might be somewhat different from that done by video assessment. We thought that parents would likely base their assessment on what the child can and does do in daily life, which might differ from the child's performance during the assessment. Furthermore parent attention might not be focused on the changes in function expected to be detected by the new measure. Since the GMFM is designed to look at quantity or "how much" the child can do without "hands-on" help, it might be more difficult for parents to separate quantity from quality and assisted function.

For this correlation analysis the data were first plotted and the residuals examined to determine whether a straight line fit was appropriate. Since this was not the case, the data were transformed and a goodness-of-fit test was done before commencing the correlation

14

TABLE 3.3
Correlations between change on the GMFM-88 and change judged by parents,
therapists and "masked" video analysis

GMFM dimensions	External criterion measures		
	Therapist* (N = 136)	Parent (N = 170)	Video (N = 28)
Lying & Rolling	0.43	0.18**	0.87
Sitting	0.57	0.41	0.64
Crawling & Kneeling	0.64	0.20**	0.41
Standing	0.61	0.45	0.73
Walking, Running & Jumping	0.74	0.68	0.52
Overall	0.65	0.54	0.82

*Thirty-four children without disabilities are not included because they did not have therapists.

**It was difficult for parents whose children were functioning higher on the GMFM (*i.e.* in the standing and walking dimensions) to make judgments about change in lying and rolling areas. If only parents whose children are performing in these areas of function are included, their correlations are similar to those of therapists.

TABLE 3.4
Mean GMFM-88 change scores for children with cerebral palsy by age
and severity

Severity	<3 years	3–5 years	≥6 years
Mild	11.5	3.0	−1.4
Moderate	6.4	1.0	1.3
Severe	5.0	0.3	2.0
	F(2,29) = 2.9	F(2,35) = 0.78	F(2,38) = 2.2
	p = 0.07	p = 0.46	p = 0.13

analysis and testing for statistical significance. Statistical analysis of all data was done on a VAX 8500 computer using the statistical package SPSSX (Norusis 1986).

Changes in the total GMFM scores correlated with judgments of change made by the video-based evaluations at $r = 0.82$; with the therapists' judgments at $r = 0.65$; and with the parents' judgments at $r = 0.54$. Comparison of the three correlation coefficients gave a chi-square value of 8.35, indicating a significant difference ($p < 0.05$) between the video and parent scores. The results overall and within dimensions are presented in Table 3.3.

The *second hypothesis* postulated that after controlling for age, children with CP classified as "mild" would have a greater change in scores than those classified as "severe", with the "moderately" affected children falling between these groups. This was based on the expectation that severity of disability would be the major limiting factor in the developmental motor progress of children with CP. This hypothesis was tested using a two-way analysis of variance (clinical severity by age) (Table 3.4).

Results revealed that the amount of change in each age group was dependent on the severity of the child's disability (age × severity interaction, F[4,101] = 2.49, p<0.05). Within

TABLE 3.5
Mean GMFM-88 total scores and mean change scores for stable and
responsive groups over time (N = 127*)

	n	*First assessment*	*Second assessment*	*Change scores*
Stable group				
Overall	30	41.87	43.13	1.26
Cerebral palsy	27	35.40	36.70	1.30
Responsive group				
Overall	97	56.54	66.19	9.64
Acquired brain injury	22	56.26	71.23	14.97
Typically developing	28	58.41	61.80	11.28
Cerebral palsy	47	55.60	61.80	6.20

*Excluded from this sample are children whose parent and therapist disagreed about whether change had occurred (n = 40) and those whose parents and therapists agreed the change was negative (n = 3).

age-groups, there was no significant difference in mean change scores between the mild, moderate and severe groups. Despite an apparent trend of difference within the young group (<3 years) as hypothesized, the ANOVA result (F[2,29] = 2.9, p = 0.07) did not reach the accepted level of statistical significance, possibly due to the small sample involved in this analysis.

The *third hypothesis* stated that typically developing children under 3 years of age would show more change than typically developing children 3 years or greater. This reflects both the greater room for change in younger preschoolers, and the rapidity of quantitative motor progress in young children. This hypothesis was tested using a two-tailed Student's *t* test.

Hypothesis three was supported by a significant difference between the change scores of older and younger children without motor disabilities (*t*[29] = 4.5, p<0.001).

The *fourth hypothesis* stated that among children judged by parents and therapists as "responsive", the amount of change on the GMFM would be greatest in children recovering from acute head injury, intermediate in preschool children without motor disabilities and least in children with CP. This would be expected in view of the potentially dramatic improvements in motor function that children may demonstrate after an acute head injury that has produced severe motor dysfunction. Hypothesis four was tested using a one-way analysis of variance of change scores in the responsive group by diagnostic category (CP, ABI, TD). A Scheffé multiple comparison was done subsequently to compare differences amongst the three groups.

Hypothesis four was supported by a significant difference in change scores among children post-acute head injury (15.0%), typically developing preschoolers (11.3%), and children with CP (6.2%) (Table 3.5). Scheffé analysis revealed a significant difference between change scores for the ABI and CP groups (p<0.05).

Validating a measure for its responsiveness to change was a relatively new concept when we began to design the validation of the GMFM. The approach we chose was that proposed by Guyatt *et al.* (1987). To look at responsiveness, Guyatt proposed that one must be able to determine intra-subject variation under stable conditions as well as what would constitute a clinically important change in function.

In this study the "stable" group was considered to be those children who were identified by both parent and therapist on the five-point rating scales as "not having changed" or as "changing a tiny bit, almost the same"; similarly the "responsive" group comprised children whose parent and therapist agreed that change had occurred. It was assumed that the variability due to time in the "stable" group should be small relative to the variability due to time in the "responsive" group, if the GMFM is responsive to change and stable in the absence of change.

Clinical characteristics of stable and responsive groups

There were 30 children (17.6% of the total sample) classified by both parent and therapist as stable, and 97 (57.1%) classified as responsive. Of the remaining children, three (1.8%) were judged by both observers to have decreased in motor function. Among the remaining 40 (23.5%), parents and therapists disagreed about whether change had occurred. The mean scores on the GMFM at the first and second assessments and the mean change score for the stable and responsive groups are listed in Table 3.5.

The stable group consisted of two children with acquired brain injury, one typically developing child and 27 children with CP with a mean age of 7.2 years (SD 3 years). Sixty per cent were males. In the stable group, 65.6% were classified as "severe", 13.8% as "moderate" and 20.7% as "mild". Thirty-seven per cent of the group had a diagnosis of athetoid CP, 37% had quadriplegia, 11% had hemiplegia, 7% had diplegia, 4% had triplegia and 4% had mixed CP. Of the children with CP, 33% were considered to be mildly or moderately retarded, 26% were slow learners, and 41% were considered to be of average or above average intelligence.

The responsive group consisted of 22 children with ABI, 28 typically developing children, and 47 children with CP. Sixty per cent were males. The mean age for this group was 5.6 years (SD 5.5 years). Of the children with a diagnosis of CP, 17% were classified as "severe", 53% as "moderate" and 28% as "mild". Of the children with CP in the "responsive" group 49% had diplegia, 21% had quadriplegia, 17% had hemiplegia, 6% had mixed CP, 4% were classified as hypotonic and 2% had athetosis.

A repeated measures ANOVA on the first and second assessment scores was calculated to assess the variability in scores over time in both the stable and responsive groups. The F statistics from these two ANOVA tables were used to calculate an intraclass correlation for each group using the formula described by Kraemer and Karner (1976). It was then possible to use the Fisher z transformation and compare the two correlation coefficients to determine whether they were significantly different from each other at alpha = 0.05. When comparing the variability on the GMFM due to time in the "stable" group with variability in the "responsive" group, there was no significant difference between first and second assessments for the stable group (ICC = 0.41, p = 0.14, Fisher z = 0.43, and a significant difference for the responsive group (ICC = 0.97, p<0.0001, Fisher z = 2.09). Results showed a significant difference between the two Fisher z correlation coefficients at p<0.01.

17

TABLE 3.6
Parental judgment of the magnitude and importance* (NB) of change in gross motor function compared to the actual change in GMFM-88 score for the cerebral palsy sample (N = 108)

Judgment of magnitude of change in gross motor function	Actual mean (%) change in GMFM score	Judgment of NB* change in GMFM score
Large negative	−9.9	4.0
Medium negative	−3.7	6.0
Small negative	—	—
No change	−1.7	—
Small positive	2.7	4.6
Medium positive	5.2	5.8
Large positive	11.4	6.0

*Importance was measured on a seven-point scale ranging from 0 ("not at all important") to 7 ("tremendously important").

TABLE 3.7
Therapist judgment of the magnitude and importance* (NB) of change in gross motor function compared to the actual change in the GMFM-88 score for children with cerebral palsy (N = 108)

Judgment of magnitude of change in gross motor function	Actual mean (%) change in GMFM score	Judgment of NB* change in GMFM score
Large negative	—	—
Medium negative	−7.9	4.6
Small negative	−2.0	3.6
No change	1.3	—
Small positive	1.3	3.8
Medium positive	7.0	5.4
Large positive	24.6	6.0

*Importance was measured on a seven-point scale ranging from 0 ("not at all important") to 7 ("tremendously important").

Determining a clinically important change

Inspection of the data indicated that parent and therapist judgments of importance of the observed change showed some relationship to the actual GMFM-determined change, although the correlation was not statistically significant. These data are presented in Tables 3.6 and 3.7 as mean positive or negative changes in three categories (small, medium, large change) in relation to mean judgments of importance. Note that judgments about the magnitude of change were made on a 15-point scale from −7 ("a very great deal less") to +7 ("a very great deal more"). Subsequently the data were collapsed to reach an overall seven-category range. Importance judgments were made using a separate seven-point scale ranging from 0 ("not at all important") to 7 ("tremendously important").

Reliability

Several sources of variation may reduce the reliability of a measure. These include variation due to assessors, subjects, the environment and the measure itself. In developing the GMFM a number of steps were taken to maximize true response and minimize variability in the validation study.

(i) To reduce inter-rater variation, all physical therapists were trained to a criterion level in the use of the GMFM and were tested prior to enrolling children in the study.

(ii) To eliminate inter-rater variability in the validation study, the same physiotherapist administered the GMFM on both occasions.

(iii) To put the child at ease as much as possible, testing was usually completed by the child's "regular" therapist in a treatment room familiar to the child. Therapists kept the testing environment as consistent as possible, including the room and the time of day at which the reassessments were done.

(iv) As the GMFM is an observational instrument, an attempt was made to minimize variation by evaluating "does do" rather than "can do". The administration guidelines prohibited any "hands-on" assistance and did not require judgment of "minimal" and "maximal" assistance. By providing objective definitions of items and a standardized scoring system presented in a manual, observer variation was also minimized.

INTRA-RATER AND INTER-RATER RELIABILITY

Intra-rater and inter-rater reliabilities were calculated from test–retest conditions. Six therapists (three from each of the original centres) participated in the reliability studies. They had a mean of 6.4 years pediatric experience, varying from 2.5 to 18 years. Twelve children chosen by the therapists to represent a spectrum of age and severity of CP were included in the study. Eleven of the 12 were used for the inter-rater reliability study and 10 of the 12 for the intra-rater reliability study.

Inter-rater reliability was determined by use of the intraclass correlation coefficient between testers when each pair of testers administered and scored the GMFM on the same child within a two-week period. This method looks at the reliability between testers of administering and scoring rather than just scoring alone, as would be the case if both therapists had scored the same videotape of a child.

The intra-rater method incorporates the variability due to subjects. Even though the time frame for the retest assessment was limited to less than two weeks, when one would not expect a large true change in function, the variance is increased by any real change in the subjects' performance.

All reliabilities were calculated using intraclass correlations derived from an analysis of variance model. An intraclass correlation ≥ 0.75 was considered acceptable for all reliability coefficients.

Table 3.8 presents intra- and inter-rater reliabilities for repeated administration of the GMFM-88. All dimensions and the total score reached an acceptable level of reliability indicating that the GMFM-88 can be used very consistently by the same assessor over time and by different therapists.

TABLE 3.8
Intra- and inter-rater reliability of the GMFM-88

GMFM dimension	Intra-rater (N=10)	Inter-rater (N=11)
Lying & Rolling	0.99	0.87
Sitting	0.99	0.92
Crawling & Kneeling	0.99	0.98
Standing	0.92	0.99
Walking, Running & Jumping	0.99	0.99
Total	0.99	0.99

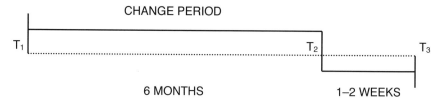

Fig. 3.1. Time line demonstrating period of study to assess reliability of observer judgments of change over time.

T_1 (time 1) = initial information on the child's motor function from standardized questionnaire.

T_2 (time 2) = judgment of change in motor function from T_1 to T_2 based on comparison with judgment at T_1.

T_3 (time 3) = judgment of change in motor function from T_1 to T_3. No true change in motor function is expected to have taken place between T_2 and T_3.

RELIABILITY OF CHANGE

The first construct validity hypothesis required the use of judgments of change by parents and therapists. It was therefore essential to assess how reliably these observers could assess change on repeated questioning. A random sample of cases (n = 23) was selected to determine how consistently change in function could be judged from one week to the next.

Each parent and physical therapist was interviewed separately on two occasions one to two weeks apart (Fig. 3.1). This interval was chosen to minimize the chance of change between the two interviews while allowing enough time so that the therapists and parents would be unlikely to remember their previous responses. On each occasion the respondent was asked to make a judgment as to whether, based on current activities, they felt that the child had changed in motor function from the time of their initial assessment (T_1). They were reminded what they had said at T_1 regarding the child's motor function and, based on that information, made a judgment as to whether change had occurred and if so, the magnitude of that change. A 15-point Likert scale varying from –7 ("a very great deal less") to +7 ("a very great deal more"), was used to quantify change. Zero represented no change.

Intra-rater reliability of estimated change scores was compared (T_1 to T_2 and T_1 to T_3). Three sources of variability enter into the reliability equation: subjects, time, and error. With an intraclass correlation of at least 0.75, it would be possible to demonstrate that at least

TABLE 3.9
Reliability of judgments of change

GMFM dimension	Therapists (n=23)	Parents (n=23)
Lying & Rolling	0.98	0.83
Sitting	0.92	0.70
Crawling & Kneeling	0.85	0.67
Standing	0.95	0.91
Walking, Running & Jumping	0.95	0.92
Total	0.96	0.92

75% of the variance was attributable to differences between subjects, with the variability between judgments at T_2 and T_3 being small.

Table 3.9 presents the reliability values for repeat judgments of change in motor function made independently by therapists and parents. With the exception of parent judgments of change in sitting and crawling and kneeling, all reliabilities of judgments of change reached acceptable levels.

Summary

Evidence from our initial validation of the GMFM-88 (Russell *et al.* 1989) has shown the GMFM-88 to be reliable, valid and responsive to change in gross motor function for children with CP. Since this initial work the evidence for the validity of the measure has grown. Bjornson *et al.* (1998b) have provided additional validation evidence of the responsiveness of the GMFM-88 for children with spastic diplegic and quadriplegic CP, and Kolobe *et al.* (1998) have established the responsiveness of the GMFM-88 for infants under 24 months of age with CP and motor delay. Palisano *et al.* (2000) used the GMFM to validate the Gross Motor Function Classification System (GMFCS) by examining the relationship between classification of severity of motor disability and gross motor function. This work adds to our confidence of the GMFM-88 as a discriminative measure as well as a responsive one. Further reliability evidence has also been established (Bjornson *et al.* 1994, 1998a; Nordmark *et al.* 1997).

The GMFM-88 has been used extensively in clinical practice and research studies to assess a variety of interventions including: physical therapy (Bower and McLellan 1992; Bower *et al.* 1996, 2001; Mulligan *et al.* 1999), rhizotomy (Salokorpi *et al.* 1997, Steinbok *et al.* 1997a, Hays *et al.* 1998, McLaughlin *et al.* 1998, Wright *et al.* 1998, Nordmark *et al.* 2000, Sacco *et al.* 2000), intrathecal baclofen (Almeida *et al.* 1997, Krach *et al.* 1997), botulinum toxin (Flett *et al.* 1999, Mall *et al.* 2000, Ubhi *et al.* 2000), pallidal stimulation (Gill *et al.* 2001), therapeutic electrical stimulation (Steinbok *et al.* 1997b), muscle tendon surgery (Abel *et al.* 1997), ambulatory aids and orthoses (Evans *et al.* 1994, Wright *et al.* 1997, Buckon *et al.* 2001, Maltais *et al.* 2001), horseback riding (MacKinnon *et al.* 1995) strength training, gait and physical fitness (MacPhail and Kramer 1995; Damiano and Abel 1996, 1998; Drouin *et al.* 1996; Harris *et al.* 1997; Campbell Torpey and Herrle 2000; Damiano *et al.* 2000; Schindl *et al.* 2000).

21

While not originally validated for children with diagnoses other than CP, the GMFM-88 has been used for other children with motor difficulties including children with osteogenesis imperfecta (Ruck-Gibis *et al.* 2001), and acute lymphoblastic leukaemia (Wright *et al.* 1998). Russell *et al.* (1998) validated the GMFM-88 for use with children with Down syndrome; however, they advocate an alternative scoring method that incorporates parent reports of activities the child can do but are not demonstrated during the assessment. For further information on administering and scoring the GMFM-88 for children with Down syndrome, see Chapter 5.

Training users on the GMFM
The GMFM was designed as a clinical assessment tool to measure change in gross motor function of children with CP. Every effort was made to ensure that the content was clinically relevant. We tried to include items that had the potential to change as a result of therapy, learning or natural development. The focus was on children's function, and particularly on motor behaviours that would be easily and consistently observable to the assessor. Response options were formulated to balance the wish for responsiveness to change in function against the challenge of limiting reliability by having too many response options. The effort we made in this respect was to try to maximize the reliability of users. Evidence from our work and the studies of others suggests that this goal has been reached successfully (Russell *et al.* 1989, 1994; Bjornson *et al.* 1994, 1998a; Nordmark *et al.* 1997).

Reliability refers to the ability of a test to give consistent results. A number of sources of variation may affect the reliability of results obtained when using a measure. These include problems with the test itself (the "examination") (*e.g.* unclear administration guidelines or a scoring system that is imprecise). Variability among assessors can arise when a user (the "examiner") is untrained, or has biases about what they should observe or how to interpret what they see. A third source of unreliability can arise when the person being assessed (the "examinee") varies from day to day when no real change has occurred (such as might happen with young children whose cooperation varies, or who perform less well in the afternoon than the morning, or are ill when assessed and do not demonstrate their best function).

Several types of reliability have been described (McDowell and Newell 1987, Streiner and Norman 1989). Obviously one wants to be sure that one's performance is accurate (consistent) when compared against an established standard; this is the type of reliability that we have been able to evaluate in the GMFM training workshops using criterion testing. One may wish to assess whether Assessor 1 and Assessor 2 are consistent in how they evaluate the same individual (inter-rater reliability), or whether assessors are consistent with themselves on repeated assessments (intra-rater reliability) or over time when the person they are assessing has not changed (test–retest reliability). These forms of reliability are important because, although it is ideal to have the same assessors evaluate the same subjects over time, this is not always possible in practice. In fact, even if it were possible to use the same assessor over time it is important to know that the assessor is using the measure in the same way from one assessment to the next, something that can be evaluated by repeat testing.

The importance of having high reliability is obvious. We need to be sure that the assessments are being done well or accurately enough that one can have confidence in the findings of a particular assessment, and be confident that variations in performance observed in clinical or research situations are due to "real" change and not to variations in the assessment process (*i.e.* poor reliability). Training users in the proper application of the GMFM has helped to ensure that those users are reliable.

In light of our interest to ensure that people used the GMFM reliably, we began to offer one-day workshops on the administration and scoring of the GMFM-88. Over the first 10 years after the GMFM was published approximately 90 workshops were held around the world, and involved over 1500 users. We took advantage of the opportunity to evaluate the effectiveness of the training programme (Russell *et al.* 1994), and to use the results of these assessments to improve the training we offered.

The approach we took was to evaluate the agreement of workshop participants with an expert scored criterion videotape pre- and post-training. A kappa statistic using a quadratic weight was used to analyse chance-corrected agreement between the rater's scoring and the criterion scoring. This kappa statistic weights disagreements so that the further away a person is from the correct score, the more they are penalized. When a weighted kappa is calculated using quadratic weights, it yields identical results to the intra-class correlation coefficient (Streiner and Norman 1989). We found that workshop participants demonstrated a statistically significant increase in agreement from a mean estimated kappa of 0.58 based on pre-workshop scores to 0.82 following a day-long workshop [$t(75) = 15.38$, $p2 < 0.001$] using one criterion testing tape, and from 0.81 to 0.92 [$t(72) = 10.91$, $p2 < 0.001$] using a second criterion testing tape (Russell *et al.* 1994). The results of this study demonstrate that clinicians who attend a one-day GMFM training workshop improve their scoring reliability significantly when tested against a criterion videotape.

As part of the data analysis for the evaluation of training effects, the number of years of pediatric neurological experience was correlated with the estimated kappa values of workshop participants ($n = 149$) to determine whether experienced clinicians were more reliable than less experienced clinicians. This was found not to be the case, with years of experience correlating at $r = -0.4$ with the pre-test values and $r = -0.1$ with the post-test values. This suggests that years of pediatric experience should not preclude people undergoing the training process.

Recently we created a CD-ROM self-training program that is based on information gained from conducting training workshops. The CD-ROM (Lane and Russell 2002) allows training to be more readily available internationally. It shows examples of several children attempting all 88 GMFM items. It allows the user to try to score each item prior to receiving feedback about the correct response. It is possible to repeat the video clips as often as needed in learning the details of how to assess each item. There is a brief introduction to the GMFM, but people who plan to learn the GMFM using the CD-ROM will need a copy of the manual in order to understand the concepts behind the measure and the details about the equipment and administration. One recent study (Lim *et al.* 2000), using an early prototype of the CD-ROM training program, has shown that people who only studied the manual performed as reliably on the criterion test as people who used the CD-ROM and manual together to learn the GMFM. The "manual only" group took significantly less time (2.75 hours vs 4.07 hours) in training. In addition to using an early version of the CD-ROM software where technical problems were still present, the authors identified that a limitation of their study was the small sample size that may have prevented them from finding a difference between the groups even if one existed (type II error). While it is possible to become a reliable user of the GMFM by reading the guidelines, feedback from people who have used the CD-ROM suggests they find the visual learning method more helpful and interesting than just reading the manual. It will be important to assess the effectiveness of the various training methods for administering and scoring the GMFM in the clinical setting using children in addition to assessing through the scoring of videotapes.

How can I assess reliability in the absence of criterion testing?
In the absence of the availability of criterion testing that has until recently been provided at GMFM training workshops, what can an individual do to develop skill in using the GMFM reliably? The first step is to read the Administration and Scoring Guidelines carefully and learn the items of the measure. Then watch the CD-ROM training program as often as necessary to become familiar with the items. People should practice using the GMFM several times prior to evaluating their reliability. Experienced GMFM users can help the new assessor with tips on the application of the measure, and can be a comparison assessor against which the new user can compare their performance. Feedback and discussion about the (mis)interpretation of items will help both the neophyte and the experienced user to become more effective assessors.

When the GMFM will be used for research purposes, a couple of strategies can be considered. It may be helpful to create criterion tapes that demonstrate the GMFM items being assessed accurately, and have criterion scores available by which to assess a new user's performance. Alternatively one can build a reliability substudy into the design of the "main" study, specifically to enable the investigators to evaluate and report on the reliability of the assessors in that specific study.

Who should use the GMFM?
We believe that, like other clinical measures, the GMFM should be used by people who are familiar and comfortable with children with disabilities, who have been trained in the use of clinical measures, and who are specifically familiar with and trained on the use of the GMFM. In general these criteria describe physical and occupational therapists who have been trained to use measures, though members of other disciplines have learned to use the GMFM reliably. It is important to recognize that measures like the GMFM differ from clinical "assessments" in being structured and standardized in an effort, as much as possible, to remove individual interpretations about performance and ensure consistency (reliability) in the application and scoring of the GMFM.

Thus, children who are noncompliant but quite high functioning may receive low scores because of their refusal to perform items that are easy for them.

An alternative approach to scoring a Rasched measure is to use a computer scoring program. This can provide summary score results that take account of not only how many items a child succeeds on, but also how difficult those items are. In addition, the use of a computer scoring system does not require that all items be tested for every subject. The CD-ROM accompanying this manual contains a user-friendly scoring program, the Gross Motor Ability Estimator (GMAE), to convert GMFM item scores into a Rasch score. The GMAE is described in more detail in Chapter 6, and the tutorial for its use is reproduced in Appendix 2.

Unlike some other health outcome measures that have been developed or modified using item response theory (*e.g.* the PEDI) there is no person-fit indicator provided with the GMFM-66. There are a number of reasons for this. First, the inclusion of item maps provides the clinician with a visual indication of the fit of the child to the underlying model of gross motor function—so while there is no quantitative means of assessing fit, it *can* be assessed qualitatively. Second, while there are a number of statistics available for analysing the person fit there is still much debate over which is the best (Molenaar and Hoijtinik 1990, Smith 1996, Li and Olejnik 1997, Smith *et al.* 1998). Finally, even though some children may respond unexpectedly to a number of items, the GMFM-66 score is still the best estimate of their ability. Refer to Appendix 9 for a discussion of two children who were identified as misfitting the model.

Reliability of the GMFM-66
Because the method of assessing GMFM items is not altered for the GMFM-66, we felt that it was not necessary to redo a study of the test–retest and inter-rater reliabilities of the 66-item GMFM. However, we did use data from a previous reliability study of the GMFM-88 to compute reliability estimates for the GMFM-66. To do this we used the GMFM-88 scores entered into the GMAE program to derive the GMFM-66 scores. The test–retest reliability results demonstrated that the GMFM-66 showed a high level of stability over time giving an intraclass correlation coefficient (ICC=0.9932) that was essentially the same reliability for the GMFM-88 (ICC=0.9944) (Russell *et al.* 2000).

RELIABILITY OF THE ITEM CALIBRATIONS AND CHILD ABILITY SCORES
In order to ensure that the item difficulty estimates and the child ability estimates were consistent, reliability analyses more specific to the Rasch method were performed. Three main issues were addressed: (i) reliability of item difficulties estimated with different samples; (ii) reliability of item difficulties over time for a single sample; (3) reliability of child scores using different items.

RELIABILITY OF ITEM DIFFICULTIES ESTIMATED WITH DIFFERENT SAMPLES
Testing the reliability of the item difficulties across samples is important to ensure the generalizability of the results. If the item ordering or the relative difficulty of the items is different for different samples then the measure is not consistent across the population of

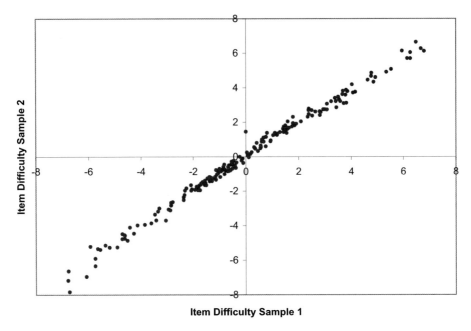

Fig. 4.3. Agreement between item step difficulty estimates obtained using two distinct samples of children.

interest and is therefore of very limited use. It should be noted that because the partial credit model makes no assumption about the relative difficulties of the steps within the items, it is necessary to satisfy the more stringent condition that item *step* difficulties are consistent when the partial credit model is used.

The reliability of item difficulties across samples was calculated by performing a Rasch analysis using two separate samples of children with CP and then comparing the resulting item step difficulties. To obtain the two samples, children in the study sample were randomly assigned to one of two groups (N = 268 per group). One child was excluded to ensure equal sample sizes in the two groups. Rasch analysis was then applied to each group's scores to obtain item difficulty estimates and item step difficulty estimates of the GMFM-66 items. Figure 4.3 illustrates the agreement of the item step difficulties between the two samples. Examination with an intra-class correlation coefficient indicated high agreement between estimates (r = 0.976, p<0.001) (Shrout and Fleiss 1979).

RELIABILITY OF ITEM DIFFICULTIES OVER TIME
To be a reliable indicator of change a measure must be consistent over time. If the relative difficulty of the items *did* change over time as a child gained or lost ability then it would be impossible to gauge a child's progress accurately. Attempting to determine the amount of change in a child using items that changed in difficulty would be like trying to determine

36

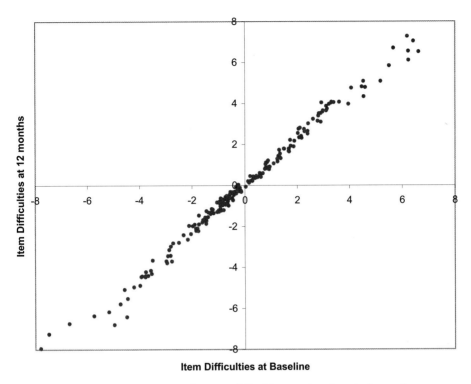

Fig. 4.4. Agreement between item step difficulties over time for a single sample.

how much a child has grown with a meter stick that can be stretched from one assessment to another.

The reliability of the item step difficulties was again examined using an intra-class correlation coefficient. However, for this analysis the comparison involved a single sample of children (N = 228) assessed 12 months apart. The baseline assessments formed one "group" on which to perform the Rasch analysis, and the assessments on the same children 12 months later formed the second group. Figure 4.4 illustrates the agreement of step difficulties over time for a single sample. Again, the intra-class correlation indicates high agreement between the difficulties (ICC = 0.966, p<0.001).

RELIABILITY OF CHILD ABILITY SCORES USING DIFFERENT ITEMS
To score the GMFM-66 it is no longer necessary to test every item in the measure. This new flexibility introduces an important question: is it possible reliably to measure change in motor function for a child if different items are tested at each assessment? To answer this question we investigated the *test-free* properties of the GMFM-66.

In order to measure the reliability of the measure across items the GMFM-66 scores were estimated twice for the study sample using separate groups of items. To obtain the two "item groups" the items were ordered by difficulty and then alternately assigned to one

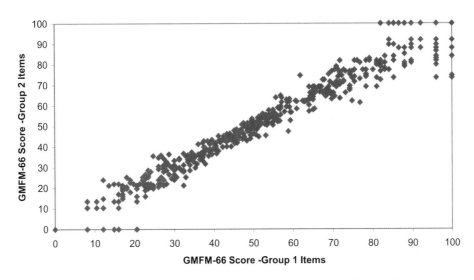

Fig. 4.5. Agreement between child ability scores using two groups of GMFM items.

of two groups (*i.e.* odd-numbered and even-numbered items). This approach was taken to ensure that each item group covered a broad range of the ability spectrum. Again, the agreement was measured using an intraclass correlation coefficient, the difference being that this analysis required the comparison of GMFM-66 scores instead of item step difficulties (Fig. 4.5). The intraclass correlation coefficient again showed significant agreement (ICC = 0.975, p<0.001).

Validity of the GMFM-66

Russell *et al.* (2000) describe in detail the evidence for reliability, validity and responsiveness of the GMFM-66. Face validity was established by examining the hierarchy of items and by examining GMFM-66 scores for different groups of children of different diagnostic types and severity levels (using the GMFCS) to see whether the outcomes made clinical sense in terms of what we know about CP.

Table 4.3 lists the hierarchy of items. Items range from the easiest, item 21: "Sit on mat supported at thorax by therapist: Lifts head upright, maintains 3 seconds", where a child with a GMFM-66 score of 24.72 would very likely have a score of 3 on that item, to the most difficult, item 80: "Stand: Jumps 30 cm (12 in) high, both feet simultaneously", where a child would need a score close to 100 to be very likely to score a 3 on that item. As one scans the list of GMFM-66 items arranged in order of difficulty, they make clinical sense.

In addition, Table 4.4 shows the distribution of GMFM-66 scores by GMFCS level and diagnostic type. There is a gradient in scores from children with relatively mild motor impairment in GMFCS level I with high GMFM-66 scores of on average 78.06, to children of comparable ages in GMFCS level V with more severe limitations and GMFM-66 scores averaging 20.63. There is also a gradient of scores by diagnostic type, with children classified

TABLE 4.4
Sample characteristics by mean GMFM-66 score and age (N=537)

	Baseline GMFM-66 score				Age at baseline				N
	Mean	SD	Min	Max	Mean	SD	Min	Max	
Type of CP									
Spastic	53.93	23.46	0.00	100.00	6.48	2.79	0.95	12.71	411
Dystonic/athetotic	37.35	14.96	17.01	67.75	5.11	2.15	1.67	9.23	32
Ataxic	60.84	11.75	41.79	74.75	6.42	2.88	2.13	10.02	14
Low tone—hypotonic	47.87	23.02	0.00	100.00	6.67	2.52	1.71	10.66	27
Mixed	40.90	21.19	0.00	100.00	6.61	2.73	1.62	11.06	53
Distribution									
Leg dominant	62.21	16.04	14.83	100.00	6.41	2.69	0.95	11.74	183
Three-limb dominant	47.80	14.67	22.66	89.70	6.63	2.45	1.81	11.06	53
Four-limb dominant	33.57	17.00	0.00	100.00	6.45	2.80	1.52	12.71	215
Right hemiplegic	75.08	15.81	43.26	100.00	6.09	3.17	1.72	11.57	43
Left hemiplegic	78.62	16.71	34.84	100.00	6.52	2.80	1.59	11.82	42
Missing	—	—	—	—	—	—	—	—	1
GMFCS level									
Level I	78.06	13.29	45.91	100.00	6.52	2.83	1.59	11.82	155
Level II	60.92	11.16	34.84	89.70	5.89	2.77	1.69	10.78	70
Level III	49.98	7.07	29.31	67.04	6.68	2.83	0.95	11.73	104
Level IV	37.94	7.77	19.72	52.85	6.38	2.63	1.62	11.74	105
Level V	20.63	8.66	0.00	46.67	6.45	2.68	1.68	12.71	103
Gender									
Male	52.04	23.85	0.00	100.00	6.38	2.84	0.95	12.71	399
Female	51.18	22.38	0.00	100.00	6.49	2.65	1.52	11.82	238

Reprinted by permission from Russell *et al.* (2000).

as having hemiplegia having the highest mean GMFM-66 scores (76.83) and children with quadriplegia the lowest (33.57).

CONSTRUCT VALIDITY AND RESPONSIVENESS OF THE GMFM-66
The GMFM was designed primarily as a measure of change. It was therefore important to ensure that the GMFM-66 was as responsive to change over time as the GMFM-88. To ensure that this responsiveness was retained, change scores for a sample of children were compared against the *a priori* hypothesis that younger children with "mild" CP would change significantly more than older children with more "severe" CP.

RESPONSIVENESS STUDY SAMPLE
All children from the original sample with two assessments 12 (±1) months apart (N = 228) were used for the responsiveness analysis. They comprised 142 males (62.3%) and 86 females: sample characteristics are shown in Tables 4.5–4.7.

RESPONSIVENESS ANALYSIS
A three-way ANOVA was performed on the GMFM-66 scores at baseline and 12 months, using severity and age as between-subject factors and time as the within-subject factor.

TABLE 4.5
Number of children by clinical distribution in the responsiveness study of the GMFM-66

Distribution	N	%
Leg dominant	74	32.5
Three-limb dominant	30	13.2
Four-limb dominant	79	34.6
Right hemiplegic	24	10.5
Left hemiplegic	18	7.9
Bilateral/double hemiplegic	3	1.3
Total	228	100.0

TABLE 4.6
Distribution of children by type of cerebral palsy in the responsiveness study of the GMFM-66

Type of CP	N	%
Spastic	173	75.9
Dystonic/athetotic	17	7.5
Ataxic	5	2.2
Low tone-hypotonic	15	6.6
Mixed	18	7.9
Total	228	100.0

TABLE 4.7
Distribution of children by severity of cerebral palsy in the responsiveness study of the GMFM-66

GMFCS level	N	%
Level I	61	26.8
Level II	35	15.3
Level III	49	21.5
Level IV	48	21.1
Level V	35	15.3
Total	228	100.0

TABLE 4.8
GMFM-66 change scores from baseline to 12 months later

GMFCS level	<5 years			5+ years		
	Mean	SD	n	Mean	SD	n
Levels I & II	7.00	4.54	39	−0.12	2.06	57
Level III	3.35	3.39	16	0.20	1.15	33
Levels IV & V	3.19	4.76	24	0.31	1.60	59
Total			79			149

Table 4.8 presents the means and standard deviations of the change scores from baseline to 12 months for the six groups of children. The results of the ANOVA show a significant Time × Age × Severity interaction [$F(2) = 12.6$, $p<0.001$]. Children under 5 years of age changed more than children over 5 years, and the greatest change was observed among the young children whose GMFCS level was level I or level II. Regardless of GMFCS level, the mean change for children over 5 years old was approximately zero even though some individual children did show both positive and negative changes.

Summary
Rasch analysis of the 88-item GMFM identified 66 of the original 88 GMFM items that met the assumptions of unidimensionality, test-free and sample-free measurement. The GMFM-66 shows good levels of reliability, validity and responsiveness. It has a hierarchical structure with interval scaling that should improve the scoring, interpretation and overall clinical utility over the GMFM-88.

5
ADMINISTRATION AND SCORING GUIDELINES FOR THE GMFM-88 AND GMFM-66

Overview

The GMFM is a standardized observational instrument that has been designed to measure change in gross motor function over time in children with cerebral palsy (CP). It was developed for use in both clinical and research settings. The first part of this chapter deals with the administration and scoring for children with CP including a section on the use of the GMFM-88 to assess aids and orthoses. There is a section on administering and scoring the GMFM-66 that is to be used only for children with CP.

Validation of the GMFM-88 for use with children with Down syndrome (DS) has also been completed. While much of the administration and scoring of the GMFM-88 is the same for children with DS, there are differences that are highlighted in this chapter.

The revised GMFM-88 and 66 scoresheet, the scoring guidelines for individual items and the explanation of terms are found near the end of this chapter.

The GMFM is designed to assess how much of an item a child can accomplish rather than measure how well the activity is performed.

The original GMFM consisted of 88 items, grouped into five different dimensions of gross motor function: Lying & Rolling; Sitting; Crawling & Kneeling; Standing; Walking, Running & Jumping. It is expected that all 88 items can be completed by a 5-year-old child without motor impairments.

Since the development of the original GMFM, extensive further work (described in this manual) has been done to validate the GMFM-66, a version of the measure that has been created using Rasch analysis to produce an interval scale. The administration of the GMFM is the same for both versions of the measure; however, there are some differences with respect to how many items are required to be tested, how the assessor scores items that are refused or not tested, and how the data are analysed once they have been collected.

The instructions described in this chapter and a GMFM scoresheet are necessary for administering this test.

Examiner qualifications

The GMFM is designed for use by pediatric therapists. The exact type and amount of formal training in the use of the measure that is necessary to ensure competency is yet to be determined. However, results from the evaluation of GMFM training workshops have shown that participants significantly improve their scoring agreement with a criterion test videotape following training (Russell *et al.* 1994).

Before assessing children, users should familiarize themselves with the scoresheet and the administration and scoring guidelines contained in this chapter, to ensure accuracy and consistency. At least two children should be tested as a practice exercise, and ideally users should check their reliability with several colleagues before employing the GMFM for clinical assessment or research purposes. A self-instructional GMFM training CD-ROM has been developed based on experience from training workshops (Lane and Russell 2002).

Time required
The time required to complete the GMFM-88 is approximately 45–60 minutes. Some children may find it too tiring to complete the full test in one session or become non-compliant for a variety of reasons. For these children it may be necessary to use more than one session or use the GMFM-66. However, any item completed in one session should not be retested in another session. It is suggested that the GMFM-88 be completed within one week to avoid changes in scoring that could be attributed to a change in the children's functional level during the assessment period. The GMFM-66 requires 22 fewer items to be administered, and the scoring program for the GMFM-66 can allow for some missing data (items that are not tested), so that it should require less time to administer.

General administration guidelines
EQUIPMENT
All necessary equipment should be assembled ahead of time and adjusted to the appropriate heights. The floor should be marked with two clearly identified straight parallel lines (taped or painted), 6 m (20 ft) long and spaced 20 cm (8 in) apart, with one of these lines 2 cm (¾ in) wide. A 60 cm (24 in) diameter circle should be marked in the same manner.

All items in Lying & Rolling, Sitting and Crawling & Kneeling are done on a mat. All items in Standing and Walking, Running & Jumping are done on the floor, with the exception of items 52, 60, 61 and 62, which may also be done on the mat.

The equipment should comprise:
- floor—smooth firm surface
- two straight lines, 20 cm (8 in) apart and 6 m (20 ft) long
- straight line, 2 cm (¾ in) wide and 6 m (20 ft) long
- circle, 60 cm (24 in) diameter marked on floor
- large firm exercise mat, minimum 1.2 × 2.4 m (4 × 8 ft) with a maximum thickness of 2.5 cm (1 in)
- small interesting toy or toys less than 10 cm (4 in) in height that can be touched with one or both hands
- small bench not longer than 1 m (3 ft) (when sitting, the child's feet should be on the floor)
- large bench (or table) appropriate in height for standing and cruising items (a rail or parallel bars may also be used)
- stopwatch or watch with a second hand
- a 30–60 cm (12–24 in) long stick for item 75
- other toys may be used to motivate the child throughout the assessment

- a larger object or toy that must be carried with two hands (*e.g.* a soccer-sized ball) for item 72
- five steps, standard rise [ca. 15 cm (6 in)] with railing
- a stool on castors may be necessary in item 51, if the child can walk forward holding on.

If any of this equipment is not available, choose equipment that is as close as possible to the specifications. Note any substitutions in equipment on the front of the score sheet under "Testing Conditions". Replicate the substitutions on subsequent testing.

ENVIRONMENT

The environment should encourage the child to demonstrate the best possible effort for each item attempted. The room should be large enough to comfortably accommodate the required equipment, child and examiner. It should be warm enough for the child to be comfortable. The floor should be a smooth firm surface. The child should feel at ease during the testing and if appropriate should be accompanied by a parent or caregiver. However, the caregiver should not help the child with any items. The tester should ensure that the testing conditions are as comfortable and as consistent as possible in order to minimize changes in scores resulting from a variation in the environment. Any specific modifications to the environment should be noted on the front of the score sheet to be certain that these are duplicated during retesting.

CLOTHING

The child should be clothed in as little as possible to allow for the examiner's unobstructed observation. Shorts and a T-shirt are ideal. The child is to be tested *without* shoes on.

TESTING

Assemble the Specific Guidelines for Item Scoring, the Explanation of Terms and the Score Sheet before starting to test. The front page of the scoresheet should be completed before testing is initiated.

Severity should be evaluated using the Gross Motor Function Classification System (GMFCS) for cerebral palsy (Palisano *et al.* 1997). This will facilitate communication and be useful for building a database of information about expected change in children of different diagnoses, ages and severities. See Appendix 1 for a detailed description of the GMFCS.

Testing conditions include any specific factors in the environment that appear to influence the child's ability to complete the measure or interfere with standardized test conditions.

It is recommended that if you are testing the GMFM-88 the items be tested in the order given and that each dimension be tested before another is initiated to avoid accidentally omitting any items.

Any item that would be feasible for the child to attempt must be tested. Although the items in each dimension are arranged approximately in a developmental sequence, we know from the Rasch analysis that items are not arranged in order of difficulty. Therefore, it cannot be assumed that any items can be scored based on the scores achieved on subsequent items. Both the dimensions and the items within the dimensions are arranged in a developmental sequence, and items at the end of one dimension may be more difficult than the items at the beginning of the next. It is therefore suggested for the GMFM-88 that items at the beginning of each dimension be tested when feasible.

It is acceptable to test items in any order. For example, if compliance is an issue, it may be advisable to begin in a dimension that is most acceptable to the child.

The child is allowed a maximum of three attempts or trials for each item. The spontaneous performance of any item is acceptable and is included as one of the three trials. The score assigned is based on the *best* performance over a maximum of three trials. If the child achieves the task in the first trial, no subsequent testing of the item is needed. Verbal encouragement or demonstration of any test item is permitted. The child may also be assisted through a "test trial" to ensure that s/he understands the item.

If necessary, the child may be placed in the starting position. As this is an observational instrument, no additional "hands-on" assistance or facilitation is permitted unless specifically indicated.

Factors that may interfere with the validity of the scores

Many children become non-compliant as soon as they sense the structure of an assessment. For these children it is suggested that as many items as possible be scored based on spontaneous performance observed within the testing environment. Any strategy that meets the defined testing guidelines can be used (*e.g.* "Follow the leader", role playing, etc.). Other toys or equipment may also be used as incentives. For example, children who are 4-point crawling often resist attempting item 38 (Prone: Creeps forward 1.8 m), even though they are able to creep. Setting up a tunnel is a very acceptable method of testing this item (especially if the child has someone to follow).

If it is believed that the child is capable of performing an item that s/he refuses to attempt, return to that item at the end of the measure. If the assessor is unable to elicit a response from the child or the child is not performing in a manner reflective of the child's typical abilities, it would be advisable to schedule another testing session or circle "not tested" (NT) for those particular items on the scoresheet.

Any item that the child does not attempt or is omitted during the assessment must be scored as "not tested". Precautions should be taken to ensure that the scores assigned reflect the child's true functional level as accurately as possible. For the GMFM-88 the items marked NT will be scored as a 0, while the GMFM-66 program will treat them as missing information.

Specific scoring administration guidelines for children with cerebral palsy

Please note that this scoring section has been modified slightly from the original GMFM scoring in order to allow both the GMFM-88 and the GMFM-66 to be used. The primary difference is the addition of the "not tested" (NT) category.

SCORING SINGLE ITEMS
Scoring is based on a four-point scale for each item using the following key:

0 = does not initiate
1 = initiates
2 = partially completes
3 = completes
NT = not tested

The scoring key is provided as a general guideline. "Does not initiate" (0) applies to the child who is requested to attempt an item and is unable to commence any part of the activity. "Initiates" (1) refers to less than 10% task completion. "Partially completes" (2) refers to a child performing from 10% to less than 100% task completion. "Completes" (3) describes 100% task completion. "Not tested" should be used when an item has not been administered or when a child refuses to attempt an item and you have reason to believe they may be able to at least partially complete it. For example an item may be difficult to elicit because the child has moved beyond it developmentally.

It is imperative that the guidelines be used for scoring each item.

For each item the starting position is always defined preceding the colon (*e.g.* item 8, Supine: Rolls to prone over right side). In this case the starting position is supine, and the remainder of the description following the colon is the maximum level of function to be achieved for that item (a score of 3).

Descriptions of the behaviours for each score (0, 1, 2, 3) are included under the description of each item in the guidelines.

The starting position is constant for each item regardless of the score they achieve, with the exception of items 48, 49 and 50. In these three items, the assessor is instructed to place the child in the required positions (for a score of 1) if the child is unable to independently attain this position.

There are two basic types of items, dynamic and static. *Dynamic* items require movement. This may include a transitional movement from one position to another (*e.g.* #14, Prone: Rolls to supine over right side) or movement while maintaining a position (*e.g.* #78, Standing: kicks ball with right foot). For the child to achieve any score beyond zero, there must be *movement* observed. *Static* items do not require movement. They require that the starting position be maintained for a specified length of time (*e.g.* #39, 4 Point: Maintains, weight on hands and knees, 10 seconds). When a score of 1 is described as "maintains <3 seconds" (*e.g.* #39) that score is intended to include those children who can maintain the position even momentarily. However, there must be some observable evidence that the child is attempting to maintain the position.

Some items involve a *combination* of both dynamic and static motor behaviour (*e.g.* item 48, Sitting on mat: Attains high kneeling using arms, maintains, arms free, 10 seconds). These all require both assuming a position and maintaining it for a specified length of time.

If undecided about what score to assign, choose the *lower* of the two possible scores.

It is very important that the child be encouraged to attempt as many items as possible to ensure that the best possible total score for each dimension is achieved.

Any item that has been omitted or that the child is unable (or unwilling) to attempt must be indicated as "not tested" (NT).

The child is allowed a maximum of three trials for each item. Remember that spontaneous

55. STD:	0 __	1 ✓	2 __	3 __	55.
56. STD:	0 ✓	1 __	2 A	3 __	56.
57. STD:	0 ✓	1 A	2 __	3 __	57.
58. STD:	0 ✓	1 A	2 __	3 __	58.
59. SIT ON SMALL BENCH:	0 __	1 ✓	2 __	3 A	59.
60. HIGH KN:	0 ✓	1 A	2 __	3 __	60.
61. HIGH KN:	0 ✓	1 A	2 __	3 __	61.
62. STD:	0 ✓	1 A	2 __	3 __	62.
63. STD:	0 ✓	1 A	2 __	3 __	63.
64. STD:	0 ✓	1 A	2 __	3 __	64.

TOTAL DIMENSION D

The Total Raw Score for Dimension D (unaided) is 7.

The Total Raw Score for Dimension D with aids/orthoses is 20.

Administering and scoring the GMFM-88 with children with Down syndrome (DS)

The GMFM-88 has been validated to measure change in gross motor function over time in children with DS (Russell *et al.* 1998). The GMFM-66 is *not* an appropriate measure for children with DS because the difficulty of GMFM-66 items was determined specifically from a large sample of children with CP and the weighting of items may be quite different for children with DS. The GMFM-88 may be used to assess children with DS; however, the authors have demonstrated that the use of "reported scores" gives better evidence of reliability, validity and responsiveness than the standard scoring approach. Guidelines for using reported scores will be discussed later in this section.

Children with DS frequently require different strategies for both assessment and treatment from those one would use for children with CP. Gemus *et al.* (2001) report on their clinical experiences using the GMFM-88 to evaluate motor function in children with DS and provide strategies they found helpful in enhancing a child's adherence to standardized testing. Those strategies are incorporated into the following guidelines.

ISSUES REGARDING EXAMINATION OF CHILDREN WITH DS

Children with DS are often more mobile than children of the same age with CP. As well, they usually have not had the same exposure to a physiotherapy environment and therefore do not have the same comfort level with physical assessment. Assessors need to be aware of these issues, as well as others related to information processing that will be described in this chapter, when planning the assessment. Assessors need to be ready to adapt both the environment and their own strategies to obtain the most complete assessment possible, and should know the items in the GMFM well enough to be able to switch items or dimensions quickly when necessary.

TIME REQUIRED

This should be the same as for children with CP. However, there may be more need for short breaks during a session or for breaking the assessment into more than one session. The same rules as described for children with CP apply if more than one session is required.

Equipment

This is the same as for children with CP. However, for children who are not used to the therapy environment the equipment used should be as familiar as possible (*i.e.* as non-institutional as possible). It may also be appropriate to have the parent bring small items that provide familiarity and comfort for the child and can be used during the assessment.

Environment

The environment should be set up the same as for children with CP. However, special emphasis should be placed on being able to control the environment and make it as free of distractions as possible. For children with good independent mobility choose a room with a door that the child can't open, and remove items that won't be required for the assessment. The room does not need to be any larger than what is required for those items that will be included in the assessment. The walking and running items require the most space. These could be done in a larger room separately from many of the other items.

Particular consideration should be given to the presence or absence of one of the child's caregivers. If reported scores are to be included, the caregiver who is most knowledgeable about the child's motor function must be present during the assessment.

Many children with DS respond best to visual rather than auditory instruction. A caregiver or other familiar person (older siblings can be helpful for this) can be very valuable in providing a role model for playing "follow the leader" with many of the GMFM items. Obviously this needs to be discussed prior to the assessment in order for these important people to be present.

Clothing

This is also the same as for children with CP. The child should be clothed in as little as possible to allow for the examiner's unobstructed observation. Shorts and a T-shirt are ideal. The child is to be tested *without* shoes on.

Testing

The guidelines for assessing children with CP on the GMFM-88 are also valid for children with DS. However, more consideration may be required before the assessment regarding who will be present and how the assessment will be structured to get the best possible result.

For children with DS, severity *cannot* be judged using the Gross Motor Function Classification System. Severity may be judged by taking muscle tone as well as gross motor competence into consideration. Table 5.1 is the motor impairment rating scale (Palisano *et al.* 2001) developed and used for the validation study of the GMFM-88 for children with DS. It is important to note, however, that further validation of the classification system is required.

Although it is easiest for the assessor to test the items in the order given, this is not likely to be what the child wants! If appropriate, give the child and caregiver a brief description of what will happen while they are with you. It is usually best to begin in the dimensions

TABLE 5.1
Motor impairment rating scale for children with Down syndrome (DS)*

Mild	Movement patterns at a similar stage of motor development are fairly typical of children without DS. The child demonstrates sufficient muscle tone, strength and voluntary control to initiate, adapt and sustain movements during play
Moderate	The child is able to initiate, adapt and sustain movements during play; however, movement patterns are less efficient compared with children without DS. The child's movements are characterized by excessive motion in some weight-bearing joints, a wide base of support, reduced balance, and compensatory movements when muscle tone and strength are not adequate to meet the demands of a task
Severe	The child has difficulty initiating, adapting and sustaining movements during play. Frequency of movement and physical endurance may be limited. Movement patterns are inefficient and characterized by compensations that reflect low muscle tone, reduced strength, and limitations in voluntary control of movement

*Adapted by permission from Palisano *et al.* (2001).

in which the child feels most comfortable or competent. It often helps to let the older child choose a dimension or group of items. However, don't get caught by asking questions that require a yes/no answer as this allows the child to refuse activities that are part of the assessment.

Children frequently will perform many items spontaneously, particularly if the room has been well prepared with appropriate equipment and toys placed to encourage the performance of activities. It is not uncommon to obtain more than half of the assessment without ever having to intervene actively with or handle the child. However, the assessor must know the measure well and be able to recognize the items and score them when they happen. A combination of spontaneous performance for as many items as possible and more specific modeling or instructions for the remaining items works well for both assessor and child. Imitation tends to be most successful with verbal instruction kept to a minimum. Both of these can be done in a very non-threatening manner especially if the caregiver or another familiar adult can be involved as well. This approach gives the assessor time to score and prepare for the next items, and the child some sense of control and enjoyment.

SPECIFIC SCORING ADMINISTRATION GUIDELINES FOR CHILDREN WITH DS
Scoring single items
The guidelines for scoring children with CP on the GMFM-88 are also valid for children with DS. Again, it is not appropriate to use the GMFM-66 for children with DS as the difficulty estimates are based on children with CP and are likely different for children with DS.

Scoring items automatically
For children with DS there are certain situations where the following items can be scored automatically. This is not applicable to children with CP.

• *Sitting: Items 21, 22, 23 and 24.* If the child is observed to maintain sit spontaneously with arms free for longer than 5 seconds you may assign a score of 3 for both items 23 and

24. You may also assign a score of 3 for items 21 and 22 if they meet the criteria for upright and/or midline. However, if the child is not observed to meet the criteria for head at midline and/or upright during this spontaneous sitting you cannot assign scores of 3 and should structure these two items as described in the guidelines to ensure that you are assigning the appropriate scores.

• *Crawling & Kneeling: Items 44 and 45.* If the child is observed to crawl forward reciprocally for 1.8 m (6 ft) you can assign a score of 3 for both item 44 and 45. If the child uses a mixture of reciprocal crawling and some form of hitching for 1.8 m (6 ft) you may assign a score of 3 for item 44 and credit item 45 only for the distance that is achieved each time there is reciprocal crawling.

You cannot credit *item 38* if the child crawls 1.8 m (6 ft).

• *Standing: Items 53 and 56 as well as 54, 55 and 57, 58.* If the child is observed to maintain stand spontaneously for at least 3 seconds you can automatically assign a score of 3 for item 53 and a score of 2 for item 56. You can then structure your testing for item 56 to see if the child can meet the criterion for a score of 3 (*i.e.* 20 secs).

If the child is observed to obtain at least a score of 2 in items 57 and/or 58 you can automatically assign a score of 3 in items 54 and/or 55. Please note that items 54 and 58 go together as do items 55 and 57.

• *Walking, Running & Jumping: Items 67, 68, 69 and 70 as well as 84, 85 and 86, 87.* If the child is observed to walk forward at least 10 steps spontaneously you can assign a score of 3 for items 67, 68 and 69. If the child includes stopping without falling at the end of the 10 steps you can also assign a score of 1 for item 70 prior to any further structuring for scoring this item any higher.

If the child is observed to obtain a score of 3 in item 86 you can also assign a score of 3 for item 84. If the child obtains a score of less than 3 in item 86 no assumptions should be made about item 84 and it should be tested as described in the guidelines.

Similarly, if the child is observed to obtain a score of 3 in item 87 you can also assign a score of 3 for item 85. If the child obtains a score of less than 3 in item 87, no assumptions should be made about item 85 and it should be tested as described in the guidelines.

Reported scores
This should be done at the time of the assessment with the caregiver who is most knowledgeable about the child's gross motor function. This can be done following the assessment (within a week), but it will be more difficult and probably less effective.

During the assessment there may be certain items that the child does not perform at all or to the level that would be expected given the scores on items of a similar or higher level of difficulty. These may be items that have been observed by the assessor or caregiver previously or that the assessor feels the child should be able to perform. For these items an "observed score" (between 0 and 2) must be assigned with a "√" based on the assessor's best effort to elicit the item. The assessor can then ask the caregiver if this is typical motor behaviour for this item outside of the assessment situation. If the caregiver says "no" then the assessor can ask the caregiver to describe what the child typically does and through careful questioning determine an appropriate reported score. This should be recorded on the score sheet with an "R". For example, in item 38 the child may be enticed to assume prone but does not creep forward more than 30 cm (1 ft) despite everyone's best efforts to encourage a distance of 1.8 m (6 ft). The caregiver is asked about the child's typical behaviour and reports having seen the child creep at least 1.8 m (6 ft) during play on the floor at home. The observed score for this item would be 1 and the reported score would be 3.

     38. PRONE: .... 0 __ 1 √ 2 __ 3 R   38.

Determining a Total Score and Goal Total Score
The GMFM-88 guidelines for children with CP are also valid for children with DS.

Determining a Total Reported Score
The calculations to determine a Total Reported Score are the same as for an observed score. For items where there is a reported score, include this score (marked with "R") in the total scores instead of the observed score (marked with a "√"). Where the item score does not have a reported score include the observed score. For example, a child may obtain the following scores for Crawling & Kneeling:

    38. PRONE: .... 0 __ 1 √ 2 __ 3 R   38.
    39. 4 POINT: .... 0 __ 1 √ 2 __ 3 R   39.
    40. 4 POINT: .... 0 __ 1 __ 2 __ 3 √   40.
    41. PRONE: .... 0 __ 1 __ 2 __ 3 √   41.
    42. 4 POINT: .... 0 __ 1 __ 2 √ 3 __   42.
    43. 4 POINT: .... 0 __ 1 __ 2 __ 3 √   43.
    44. 4 POINT: .... 0 __ 1 __ 2 __ 3 √   44.
    45. 4 POINT: .... 0 __ 1 __ 2 __ 3 √   45.
    46. 4 POINT: .... 0 __ 1 __ 2 __ 3 √   46.
    47. 4 POINT: .... 0 √ 1 R 2 __ 3 __   47.
    48. SIT ON MAT: .... 0 √ 1 __ 2 R 3 __   48.
    49. HIGH KN: .... 0 √ 1 __ 2 __ 3 __   49.
    50. HIGH KN: .... 0 √ 1 __ 2 __ 3 __   50.
    51. HIGH KN: .... 0 √ 1 __ 2 __ 3 __   51.

TOTAL DIMENSION C
The Total Raw Score for Dimension C (observed) is 22.
The Total Raw Score for Dimension C (reported) is 29.

GMFM-88 AND GMFM-66 ITEM SCORING GUIDELINES

The items for the GMFM-88 and the GMFM-66 are described in detail in this section. The GMFM-66 uses a subset of the original 88 items, which are indicated here and on the score sheet with an asterisk (*).

For the convenience of users needing to refer to these guidelines while conducting testing, they have been set in a larger type size.

LYING & ROLLING

This dimension includes 17 items in the prone and supine positions. These items include the child's ability to:
- roll from prone or supine
- perform specific tasks while maintaining supine or some variation of prone.

The following terms employed in this dimension are defined in the Explanation of Terms at the end of this chapter (pp 124–129) and/or in the item(s) in which they occur as part of the instructions. They are listed in the order in which they appear:
- supine
- asymmetrical
- fingers one with the other
- brings hands to front of body
- initiates neck flexion
- full range of hip and knee flexion
- prone
- lifts head upright
- fully extends opposite arm forward
- opposite arm comes free.

1. <u>Supine, head in midline: Turns head with extremities symmetrical</u>

    0. does not maintain head in midline
    1. maintains head in midline 1–3 seconds
    2. maintains head in midline, turns head with extremities asymmetrical
    3. turns head with extremities symmetrical

Position the child with head in midline and, if possible, the arms at rest and symmetrical (but not necessarily at the side). This will make it easier to determine the appropriate score.

INSTRUCTIONS
Instruct the child to turn the head from side to side or follow an object from one side to the other.

The child can be instructed to keep the arms still or, in the case of a younger child who may try to reach for the object, observe whether the upper extremity movements are "symmetrical" or "asymmetrical". This can be difficult to determine, particularly on videotape. For example, if you see marked asymmetry in the upper extremities and no change in the lower extremities when the child is following the toy from side to side it is quite likely that the child is simply reaching out for the toy. This child would probably meet the criterion for a score of 3.

For a score of 2 (extremities "asymmetrical") there should be very obvious asymmetry that is dominated by head position.

*2. Supine: Brings hands to midline, fingers one with the other

      0. does not initiate bilateral hands to midline
      1. initiates bilateral hands to midline
      2. brings hands to front of body, does not finger one with the other
      3. brings hands to midline, fingers one with the other

STARTING POSITION
Position the child in supine, preferably with the head in midline and arms at rest.

INSTRUCTIONS
Instruct the child to bring the hands together or to imitate your demonstration. Younger children will frequently bring hands together spontaneously especially in anticipation of a toy presented to them.

"Fingers one with the other" indicates that the child must sustain both hands together long enough to show some evidence of fingertip contact of at least one hand with the other (this can be as little as one finger touching the opposite hand but may not be fisted hands touching momentarily). The hands may be touching the body or reaching in space.

"Brings hands to front of body" indicates that the child brings both hands within the area in front of the body (*i.e.* between the shoulders). The hands may be touching the body or in space.

3. Supine: Lifts head 45°

      0. does not initiate neck flexion
      1. initiates neck flexion but does not lift head
      2. lifts head <45°
      3. lifts head 45°

STARTING POSITION
Position the child in supine, preferably with the head in midline.

INSTRUCTIONS
This item is easily elicited if the child understands the task and is cooperative. With younger children it may be more difficult. Try to engage their interest in a toy. Then, while still maintaining their attention on the toy, gradually move the toy toward their feet and out of sight. Hopefully they will attempt to lift their head in pursuit of the toy. Also consider pretending to pick up the child and the head may be lifted in anticipation. Frequently this item is demonstrated spontaneously.

For a score of 1, "initiates neck flexion", there must be some movement of the head toward neck flexion (*i.e.* lifting or tucking of the chin). This is an example of a dynamic item, therefore there must be movement observed in the intended direction to achieve any score beyond a zero.

4. Supine: Flexes right hip and knee through full range

      0. does not initiate right hip and knee flexion
      1. initiates right hip and knee flexion
      2. flexes right hip and knee through partial range
      3. flexes right hip and knee through full range

STARTING POSITION
Position the child in supine, preferably with head in midline and legs in comfortable extension.

INSTRUCTIONS
Older children may be asked to bring their knee(s) toward their chest. Younger children will often demonstrate this item spontaneously during play (bringing knees or feet to hand or mouth) or in anger (kicking). You may be able to entice a younger child to flex the hip(s) and knee(s) by placing an interesting toy on one or both feet.

This item is scored using the generic scoring key (*i.e.* 1 = less than 10%, etc.).

For "full range" of hip and knee flexion the child's knee(s) should touch (or almost touch) the chest (depending on the size of the child's thigh and/or abdomen) and the calf should touch the posterior aspect of the thigh.

5. <u>**Supine: Flexes left hip and knee through full range**</u>

    0. does not initiate left hip and knee flexion
    1. initiates left hip and knee flexion
    2. flexes left hip and knee through partial range
    3. flexes left hip and knee through full range

STARTING POSITION
Position the child in supine, preferably with head in midline and legs in comfortable extension.

INSTRUCTIONS
Older children may be asked to bring their knee(s) toward their chest. Younger children will often demonstrate this item spontaneously during play (bringing knees or feet to hand or mouth) or in anger (kicking). You may be able to entice a younger child to flex the hip(s) and knee(s) by placing an interesting toy on one or both feet.

This item is scored using the generic scoring key (*i.e.* 1 = less than 10%, etc.).

For "full range" of hip and knee flexion the child's knee(s) should touch (or almost touch) the chest (depending on the size of the child's thigh and/or abdomen) and the calf should touch the posterior aspect of the thigh.

*6. Supine: Reaches out with right arm, hand crosses midline toward toy

    0. does not initiate reaching toward midline
    1. initiates reaching toward midline
    2. reaches out with right arm, hand does not cross midline
    3. reaches out with right arm, hand crosses midline toward toy

STARTING POSITION
Position the child in supine, preferably with head in midline and arms at rest (any position is acceptable so long as they are not at or across midline). Position the toy at chest level within easy reach for the child but far enough off the chest that the hand will reach into space.

INSTRUCTIONS
Most children will respond to being asked to reach toward a small toy held at midline. As they do so, gradually move the toy toward their left to ensure that they cross midline with their right hand. However, the position of the toy will vary according to the child's ability.

    Many therapists have been tempted to hold the opposite arm down, which is not acceptable.

    For the child who always reaches with two hands or the closest hand, use a larger toy. Pass the toy from the child's right to left trying to engage both arms in reaching (the hands may not be touching one another) and hopefully achieve the goal of the right hand crossing midline.

*7. Supine: Reaches out with left arm, hand crosses midline to touch toy

    0. does not initiate reaching toward midline
    1. initiates reaching toward midline
    2. reaches out with left arm, hand does not cross midline
    3. reaches out with left arm, hand crosses midline to touch toy

STARTING POSITION
Position the child in supine preferably with head in midline and arms at rest (any position is acceptable so long as they are not at or across midline). Position the toy at chest level within easy reach for the child but far enough off the chest that the hand will reach into space.

INSTRUCTIONS

Most children will respond to being asked to reach toward a small toy held at midline. As they do so, gradually move the toy toward their right to ensure that they cross midline with their left hand. However, the position of the toy will vary according to the child's ability.

Many therapists have been tempted to hold the opposite arm down, which is not acceptable.

For the child who always reaches with two hands or the closest hand, use a larger toy. Pass the toy from the child's left to right trying to engage both arms in reaching (the hands may not be touching one another) and hopefully achieve the goal of the left hand crossing midline.

8. Supine: Rolls to prone over right side

0. does not initiate rolling
1. initiates rolling
2. rolls part way to prone
3. rolls to prone over right side

STARTING POSITION

Position the child in supine, preferably with head in midline and arms and legs comfortably at rest.

INSTRUCTIONS

With older children simply ask them to roll onto their stomach. Younger children will usually roll toward a toy.

This item uses the generic scoring key (*i.e.* 1 = less than 10%, etc.). Be careful to credit any attempt that includes movement in the direction one would anticipate for rolling to the right.

If the child rolls completely to prone but the right arm stays trapped underneath, a score of 3 may be given.

9. Supine: Rolls to prone over left side

    0. does not initiate rolling
    1. initiates rolling
    2. rolls part way to prone
    3. rolls to prone over left side

STARTING POSITION
Position the child in supine, preferably with head in midline and arms and legs comfortably at rest.

INSTRUCTIONS
With older children simply ask them to roll onto their stomach. Younger children will usually roll toward a toy.

This item uses the generic scoring key (*i.e.* 1 = less than 10%, etc.). Be careful to credit any attempt that includes movement in the direction one would anticipate for rolling to the left.

If the child rolls completely to prone but the left arm stays trapped underneath, a score of 3 may be given.

*10. Prone: Lifts head upright

    0. does not initiate head lifting
    1. initiates head lifting, chin does not clear mat
    2. lifts head, does not attain upright, chin clears mat
    3. lifts head upright

STARTING POSITION
Position the child in prone with head on the mat and arms and legs comfortably positioned (abdomen and pelvis must be in contact with the mat). The head may be face down or turned to either side.

This item is intended to include even the more severely involved (or immature) children who will attempt to lift their head when in prone.

By allowing the arms to be in any position a broad spectrum of children are included (including those who are more competent and automatically lift their head upright with weight on forearms).

INSTRUCTIONS

Older children may be asked to lift the head and look forward. Younger children may be tested by having someone in front of them to attract their attention with a toy or to call them by name.

"Lifts head upright" indicates that the head has reached vertical. It applies to the sagittal plane only (*i.e.* the eyes are forward but not necessarily horizontal).

Children who lift the head (or attempt to) while it is still turned to the side may meet the criteria for a score of 1 or 2 (depending on whether or not the child's chin clears the mat).

Children who tilt or turn the head slightly to either side but still meet the criteria for "upright" should be given a score of 3.

11. **Prone on forearms: Lifts head upright, elbows extended, chest raised**

    0. does not initiate head lifting
    1. initiates head lifting, chin does not clear mat
    2. lifts head, does not attain upright, weight on forearms
    3. lifts head upright, elbows extended, chest raised

STARTING POSITION

Position the child in prone with arms positioned for forearm weight bearing and legs in comfortable extension. The head should be on the mat if you anticipate difficulty with head lifting. Otherwise, it may be off the mat.

INSTRUCTIONS

The child is to be encouraged to lift the head to vertical and extend the arms. Older children may respond to verbal request or demonstration. Younger children are more likely to respond to a toy held in front of them and gradually elevated.

Although a score of 2 can be achieved by children who can lift the head to less than vertical with weight on forearms, it must also include children who lift the head to (or beyond) vertical but still have weight on forearms.

To obtain a score of 3 the head must be upright, the elbows must be extended enough that they are off the mat, weight must be on the hands, and the chest must be off the mat.

Children who lift the pelvis off the mat especially as they extend their arms would only be scored based on what they achieve before the pelvis is lifted.

12. Prone on forearms: Weight on right forearm, fully extends opposite arm forward

   0. does not initiate supporting weight on right forearm
   1. weight on right forearm, opposite arm comes free, does not extend forward
   2. weight on right forearm, partially extends opposite arm forward
   3. weight on right forearm, fully extends opposite arm forward

STARTING POSITION
Position the child in prone with arms positioned for forearm weight bearing and legs in comfortable extension. The head may be in any position.

INSTRUCTIONS
Place a toy at arm's length in front of the child approximately at eye level (*i.e.* approximately 15 cm (6 in) off the mat). Offer encouragement to reach forward and off the mat toward the toy with the left arm.

"Fully extends opposite arm forward" implies that the child reaches forward with the left arm off the mat into full elbow extension and forward shoulder flexion. The child who only partially extends the arm forward would be limited to a score of 2 (including those with contractures).

For a score of 1, it is stated that the "opposite arm comes free". This is intended to include any observable indication that weight is being shifted off the reaching arm with the intention of reaching forward. The arm does not need to lift off the mat, although it may.

For a score of 2, "partially extends opposite arm forward", the reaching arm still does not have to be off the mat.

For a score of 3, "fully extends opposite arm forward", the reaching arm must be off the mat.

The position of the weight-bearing arm is not critical as long as it is in contact with the mat and observed to be bearing weight (frequently it will be across the chest).

13. **Prone on forearms: Weight on left forearm, fully extends opposite arm forward**

    0. does not initiate supporting weight on left forearm
    1. weight on left forearm, opposite arm comes free, does not extend forward
    2. weight on left forearm, partially extends opposite arm forward
    3. weight on left forearm, fully extends opposite arm forward

STARTING POSITION
Position the child in prone with arms positioned for forearm weight bearing and legs in comfortable extension. The head may be in any position.

INSTRUCTIONS
Place a toy at arm's length in front of the child approximately at eye level (*i.e.* approximately 15 cm (6 in) off the mat). Offer encouragement to reach forward and off the mat toward the toy with the right arm.

"Fully extends opposite arm forward" implies that the child reaches forward with the right arm off the mat into full elbow extension and forward shoulder flexion. The child who only partially extends the arm forward would be limited to a score of 2 (including those with contractures).

For a score of 1, it is stated that the "opposite arm comes free". This is intended to include any observable indication that weight is being shifted off the reaching arm with the intention of reaching forward. The arm does not need to lift off the mat, although it may.

For a score of 2, "partially extends opposite arm forward", the reaching arm still does not have to be off the mat.

For a score of 3, "fully extend opposite arm forward", the reaching arm must be off the mat.

The position of the weight-bearing arm is not critical as long as it is in contact with the mat and observed to be bearing weight (frequently it will be across the chest).

14. Prone: Rolls to supine over right side

    0. does not initiate rolling
    1. initiates rolling
    2. rolls part way to supine
    3. rolls to supine over right side

STARTING POSITION
Position the child in prone with arms and legs comfortably positioned and preferably with head down.

INSTRUCTIONS
Encourage the child to roll to supine over the right side either by request or following demonstration. The younger child may respond to rolling toward toys or a caregiver.

It is not acceptable to position the arms so that any effort results in the child "falling" into supine without any head lifting (*e.g.* placing the right arm flexed under the head).

This item uses the generic scoring key (*i.e.* 1 = less than 10%, etc.). Remember to credit any attempt that includes movement in the direction one would anticipate for rolling to the right.

If the child rolls completely to supine but the feet remain crossed, a score of 3 should be given.

15. Prone: Rolls to supine over left side

    0. does not initiate rolling
    1. initiates rolling
    2. rolls part way to supine
    3. rolls to supine over left side

STARTING POSITION
Position the child in prone with arms and legs comfortably positioned and preferably with head down.

INSTRUCTIONS
Encourage the child to roll to supine over the left side either by request or

following demonstration. The younger child may respond to rolling toward toys or a caregiver.

It is not acceptable to position the arms so that any effort results in the child "falling" into supine with any head lifting (*e.g.* placing the left arm flexed under the head).

This item uses the generic scoring key (*i.e.* 1 = less than 10%, etc.). Remember to credit any attempt that includes movement in the direction one would anticipate for rolling to the left. If the child rolls completely to supine but the feet remain crossed, a score of 3 should be given.

16. Prone: Pivots to right 90° using extremities

0. does not initiate pivot to right
1. initiates pivot to right using extremities
2. pivots to right <90° using extremities
3. pivots to right 90° using extremities

STARTING POSITION
Position the child comfortably in prone preferably with head down.

INSTRUCTIONS
Position the toy on the child's right and offer encouragement to pivot toward it. If you suspect that the child will pivot 90° place the toy beyond 90°.

With the toy at 90° some children tend to pivot part way, then reach out for the toy with their right hand and assume they have completed the task.

The use of any combination of extremities is acceptable as long as they remain in prone.

Many children will choose to roll or crawl rather than pivot. In this case it may be preferable to begin with the toy just to the child's right and gradually move it as the child moves.

17. Prone: Pivots to left 90° using extremities

0. does not initiate pivot to left
1. initiates pivot to left using extremities
2. pivots to left <90° using extremities
3. pivots to left 90° using extremities

STARTING POSITION
Position the child comfortably in prone preferably with head down.

INSTRUCTIONS
Position the toy on the child's left and offer encouragement to pivot toward it. If you suspect that the child will pivot 90°, place the toy beyond 90°.

With the toy at 90° some children tend to pivot part way and then reach out for the toy with their left hand and assume they have completed the task.

The use of any combination of extremities is acceptable as long as they remain in prone.

Many children will choose to roll or crawl rather than pivot. In this case it may be preferable to begin with the toy just to the child's left and gradually move it as the child moves.

SITTING

This dimension includes 20 items that deal with various aspects of sitting. These include the child's ability to:
• maintain various sitting positions
• assume sitting from a variety of positions or in different situations
• move from sitting into a variety of positions
• perform specific tasks while maintaining the sitting position.

"Sitting" includes any sitting position (including "W" sitting) unless otherwise described (*e.g.* item 31, "with feet in front").

Some therapists have expressed concern that "W" sitting is allowed in many items. They feel that it may be difficult to detect real change over time if the child uses "W" sitting on one occasion and sitting with feet in front on a subsequent testing. However, there has also been a lot of support to include "W" sitting as much as possible as it is often a very functional sitting position for children with CP.

If the child demonstrates a strong preference for a specific sitting position (including "W" sitting), note this in the comments section at the end of the score sheet. If it is felt to have an impact on the scoring (positive or negative), the same position can be replicated if necessary on subsequent testing.

The following terms employed in this dimension are defined in the Explanation of Terms at the end of this chapter (pp 124–129) and/or in the item(s) in which they occur as part of the instructions. They are listed in the order in which they appear:

- sitting
- head control
- "W" sit
- lifts head upright
- lifts head to midline
- arm(s) propping
- arms free
- side sitting
- with control
- crash
- 4 point
- arms assisting
- sitting, feet supported
- sitting, feet free
- on the floor.

*18. Supine, hands grasped by examiner: Pulls self to sitting with head control

    0. does not initiate head control when pulled to sitting
    1. initiates head control when pulled to sitting
    2. assists with pulling to sitting, head control present part of the time
    3. pulls self to sitting with head control

STARTING POSITION
Position the child in supine, preferably with head in midline and arms and legs in comfortable extension.

INSTRUCTIONS
The therapist should be positioned to allow enough room for the child to come to sit but at the same time be close enough to grasp the child's hands securely. With small children the therapist can be positioned to the side but with larger children it is usually necessary to straddle their legs (be careful not to stabilize their legs).

Begin by leaning forward and securely grasping the child's hands. Their elbows should be extended as much as possible to allow them to pull themselves to sit by flexing their elbows as the therapist shifts slightly backward. Children should be instructed to pull themselves up to sitting. Observe the amount of head control exhibited and how much they are participating in pulling to sitting. "Head control" is the ability to maintain the head in line with the spine or slightly forward. (Review the definition of "sitting" in the Explanation of Terms, p 124.)

To obtain a score of 3, children must do most of the pulling (it may not be possible to begin in full elbow extension and the elbows must change from relative extension to flexion). The head must be in line with the spine or slightly flexed from beginning to end.

To obtain a score of 1, children may demonstrate some attempt at head control at any time while they are being pulled to sit.

To obtain a score of 2, children must assist with pulling and demonstrate head control for part of the time. This will include many of the children who "hang on" with flexed elbows while the therapist pulls them to sit, and/or the children with some degree of head lag, especially initially.

19. Supine: Rolls to right side, attains sitting

    0. does not initiate sitting from right side lying
    1. rolls to right side, initiates sitting
    2. rolls to right side, partially attains sitting
    3. rolls to right side, attains sitting

STARTING POSITION
Position the child in supine, preferably with head in midline and arms and legs in comfortable extension.

INSTRUCTIONS
Instruct the child to attain sitting by first rolling onto the right side. Children who already use this strategy to assume sitting will easily understand this item, but for those who do not, more explanation may be required.

Many children roll to prone from supine and assume sitting. This method does not match the description for any score and the child would receive a score of zero for this item.

Once the child has rolled to the right side, this item is scored using the generic scoring key (*i.e.* 1 = less than 10%, etc.).

20. Supine: Rolls to left side, attains sitting

    0. does not initiate sitting from left side lying
    1. rolls to left side, initiates sitting
    2. rolls to left side, partially attains sitting
    3. rolls to left side, attains sitting

STARTING POSITION
Position the child in supine, preferably with head in midline and arms and legs in comfortable extension.

INSTRUCTIONS
Instruct the child to attain sitting by first rolling onto the left side. Children who already use this strategy to assume sitting will easily understand this item, but for those children who do not, more explanation may be required.

Many children roll to prone from supine and then assume sitting. This method does not match the description for any score and the child would receive a score of zero for this item.

Once the child has rolled to the right side, this item is scored using the generic scoring key (*i.e.* 1 = less than 10%, etc.).

*21. Sitting on mat, supported at thorax by therapist: Lifts head upright, maintains 3 seconds

    0. does not initiate head lift
    1. initiates head lift
    2. lifts head, does not attain upright, holds 3 seconds
    3. lifts head upright, maintains 3 seconds

STARTING POSITION
Position the child in any comfortable sitting position with the head flexed forward. "Sitting" is defined as the ability to support the body "more or less upright" with weight on the buttocks. If the child is leaning far enough in any

71

direction that propping with the arms is used, the elbow must be off the weight-bearing surface (*e.g.* bench, mat or floor). Otherwise the child would not be upright enough to be considered "sitting". As well, leaning back further than 45° from the upright position in any direction would not be considered "sitting".

INSTRUCTIONS
The therapist is to be positioned behind the child with both hands on the thorax. It is strongly advised to have a second person in front of the child holding a toy at the child's eye level. If this is not possible the use of a wall mirror may help to hold the child's attention.

Instruct the child to lift the head and look forward at the toy. The child is expected to lift the head "upright". "Upright" indicates that the head has reached vertical. It applies to the sagittal plane only (*i.e.* the eyes are forward but not necessarily horizontal).

*22. <u>Sitting on mat, supported at thorax by therapist: Lifts head to midline, maintains 10 seconds</u>

    0. does not initiate head lift
    1. initiates head lift, does not attain midline
    2. lifts head to midline, maintains <10 seconds
    3. lifts head to midline, maintains 10 seconds

STARTING POSITION
Position the child in any comfortable sitting position. The head should be flexed forward.

INSTRUCTIONS
The therapist is to be positioned behind the child with both hands on the thorax. It is strongly advised to have a second person in front of the child holding a toy at the child's eye level. If this is not possible the use of a wall mirror may help to hold the child's attention.

Instruct the child to lift the head and look forward at the toy. The child is expected to lift the head to "midline". "Midline" indicates that the head is "in the middle" or it could be said to be vertical on both the sagittal and frontal planes (*i.e.* the eyes are forward and horizontal).

*23. Sitting on mat, arm(s) propping: Maintains 5 seconds

    0. does not maintain with arm(s) propping
    1. maintains <1 second
    2. maintains 1–4 seconds
    3. maintains 5 seconds

STARTING POSITION
Position the child on the mat in any comfortable sitting position. The arms may be positioned wherever it is most advantageous for propping. This may include in front or at the side or anywhere on the body such as the thighs. Children may also prop with one arm or one arm on top of the other (*e.g.* children with hemiplegia). Because this is an observational measure, any contact of the arm(s) on the body or the mat for the purpose of maintaining upright is to be considered "propping".

INSTRUCTIONS
The therapist may be positioned wherever it is most appropriate for children to give their best effort. For younger or more involved children, the therapist should be behind the child and a second person can offer encouragement from the front. Having the child facing a mirror may also be helpful. Older children can simply be asked to maintain the position for the required time.

*24. Sitting on mat: Maintains, arms free, 3 seconds

    0. does not maintain unless both arms propping
    1. maintains, one arm propping
    2. maintains, arms free, <3 seconds
    3. maintains, arms free, 3 seconds

STARTING POSITION
Position the child on the mat in any comfortable sitting position. The arms may be in any position.

INSTRUCTIONS
The therapist may be positioned either behind or in front of the child. Many children may choose to begin with "arms propped" and then, in response to

a verbal request, or demonstration, they may lift one or both hands. Young children may begin with arms propped and then be enticed to lift one or both arms by reaching for toys held in front of them or by joining in games that involve bilateral hand movements (*e.g.* clapping). "Arms free" indicates that no weight is taken through the arms for the purpose of attaining or maintaining the sitting position (hands clapping or clasped together is permissible).

*25. <u>Sitting on mat with small toy in front: Leans forward, touches toy, re-erects without arm propping</u>

   0. does not initiate leaning forward
   1. leans forward, does not re-erect
   2. leans forward, touches toy, re-erects with arm propping
   3. leans forward, touches toy, re-erects without arm propping

STARTING POSITION
Position the child on the mat in any comfortable sitting position. The position of the arms will vary according to the ability of the child (*e.g.* to obtain a score of 3, both arms will have to be free), but the child must be reasonably stable in sitting to attempt this item.

INSTRUCTIONS
Place the toy far enough away from the child so that it is necessary to lean forward to touch it. This will depend on numerous factors (*e.g.* initial sitting alignment, range of motion of reaching arm, etc.). Allow for at least one trial to determine if the toy is within the child's reach as well as necessitating leaning forward. For most children this will be approximately between the ankles if they are sitting with their feet in front. For older children, simply ask them to touch the toy and return to sitting without leaning on the opposite arm. Younger children are more difficult to test. Choosing a larger toy to elicit "arms free" is one strategy worth trying.

*26. <u>**Sitting on mat: Touches toy placed 45° behind child's right side, returns to start**</u>

    0. does not initiate touching toy
    1. initiates reaching, does not reach behind
    2. reaches behind, does not touch toy or return to start
    3. touches toy placed 45° behind child's right side, returns to start

STARTING POSITION
Position the child on the mat in any comfortable sitting position (this may include "W" sitting). The position of the arms may vary but the child must be reasonably stable in sitting to attempt this item.

INSTRUCTIONS
Place the toy 45° behind the child's right side at a distance from the buttocks that equals the length of the child's open hand (it may be further if this helps to motivate the child, but cannot be any closer). One would expect the child to rotate to the right and touch the toy. However, many children exhibit little or no trunk rotation and still succeed in touching the toy. This is definitely acceptable for this item provided they touch it with the right hand. Older children may simply be asked to turn and touch the toy with their right hand. Typically, it is more difficult with younger children. The therapist may try passing the toy along their right side to gain their attention and then stopping at the appropriate position, anticipating that the child will attempt to reach for it. It is important to keep their attention on the toy. For a score of 2, "reaches behind", the hand must reach beyond the greater trochanter.

*27. <u>**Sitting on mat: Touches toy placed 45° behind child's left side, returns to start**</u>

    0. does not initiate touching toy
    1. initiates reaching, does not reach behind
    2. reaches behind, does not touch toy or return to start
    3. touches toy placed 45° behind child's left side, returns to start

STARTING POSITION
Position the child on the mat in any comfortable sitting position. The position

of the arms may vary but the child must be reasonably stable in sitting to attempt this item.

INSTRUCTIONS
Place the toy 45° behind the child's left side at a distance from the buttocks that equals the length of the child's open hand (it may be further if this helps to motivate the child, but cannot be any closer). One would expect the child to rotate to the left and touch the toy. However, many children exhibit little or no trunk rotation and still succeed in touching the toy. This is definitely acceptable for this item provided they touch it with the left hand. Older children may simply be asked to turn and touch the toy with their left hand. Typically, it is more difficult with young children. The therapist may try passing the toy along their left side to gain their attention and then stopping at the appropriate position, anticipating that the child will attempt to reach for it. It is important to keep their attention on the toy. For a score of 2, "reaches behind", the hand must reach beyond the greater trochanter.

28. Right side sitting: Maintains, arms free, 5 seconds

0. does not maintain right side sitting
1. maintains, both arms propping, 5 seconds
2. maintains, right arm propping, 5 seconds
3. maintains, arms free, 5 seconds

STARTING POSITION
Position the child on the mat in right side sitting (*i.e.* weight is well over the right ischium with both legs flexed to the left and both feet close to or in line with the left hip). Children may begin with both arms propped and then try to graduate to right arm propped or arms free. Remember that arms may be propped on the body or the mat. However, for this item, if they are propping on the mat, the elbow must be off the mat, otherwise it is closer to side lying than side sitting.

INSTRUCTIONS
Instruct the child to lift the left arm or both arms. Once you have established which of the three positions will be attempted, count to 5 seconds. If the child

is unable to maintain the position for 5 seconds then try at a lower level and count to 5 seconds.

The therapist may do whatever is necessary to ensure that the child is stable in the start position but must be sure that no support is offered once timing starts. Many children will respond to imitation or engage in hand games to attempt "arms free".

29. <u>Left side sitting: Maintains, arms free, 5 seconds</u>

    0. does not maintain left side sitting
    1. maintains, both arms propping, 5 seconds
    2. maintains, left arm propping, 5 seconds
    3. maintains, arms free, 5 seconds

STARTING POSITION
Position the child on the mat in left side sitting (*i.e.* weight is well over the left ischium with both legs flexed to the right and both feet close to or in line with the right hip). Children may begin with both arms propped and then try to graduate to left arm propped or arms free. Remember that arms may be propped on their own body or the mat. However, for this item, if they are propping on the mat, the elbow must be off the mat, otherwise it is closer to side lying than side sitting.

INSTRUCTIONS
Instruct the child to lift the right arm or both arms. Once you have established which of the three positions will be attempted, count to 5 seconds. If the child is unable to maintain the position for 5 seconds then try at a lower level and count to 5 seconds.

The therapist may do whatever is necessary to ensure that the child is stable in the start position but must be sure that no support is offered once timing starts. Many children will respond to imitation or engage in hand games to attempt "arms free".

*30. <u>Sitting on mat: Lowers to prone with control</u>

    0. does not initiate lowering to prone
    1. initiates lowering to prone
    2. lowers to prone, but "crashes"
    3. lowers to prone with control

STARTING POSITION
Position the child on the mat in any comfortable sitting position. As with several preceding items, the position of the arms may vary and the child must be reasonably stable in sitting to attempt this item.

INSTRUCTIONS
It is anticipated that children will use their arms to lower with control. "With control" implies that the movement is regulated or directed. Older children may simply be asked to lie down on their stomach. For those who insist on throwing themselves down (crashing) ask them to lie down carefully. Some may require demonstration.

    "Crash" is defined as "to fall, collide or collapse". It may be seen as movement that is not controlled. It is not intended to include those children who fall over accidentally and then roll to prone. Younger children may be enticed to move to prone with a toy or book. It is often very difficult to get them to prone as they frequently prefer some variation of 4 point.

*31. <u>Sitting on mat with feet in front: Attains 4 point over right side</u>

    0. does not initiate 4 point over right side
    1. initiates 4 point over right side
    2. partially attains 4 point over right side
    3. attains 4 point over right side

STARTING POSITION
Position the child on the mat in a sitting position with their legs comfortably in front of them. Note that this differs from item 30 (*i.e.* "W" sitting is not acceptable for this item).

INSTRUCTIONS
It is anticipated that children will move through some variation of right side

sitting or move forward and to the right over their right leg. It is also expected that they will accomplish this by taking weight onto their arms. It is not important whether they take weight first onto one or both forearms and then extend their arms later or if they immediately take weight onto their hands. However, they may not assume prone first and then progress to 4 point from prone (assuming 4 point from prone is assessed in item 41).

Older children may respond to verbal instruction but many will require further explanation. Demonstration or "walking them through it" may be necessary.

Young children will again need to be enticed with strategic placement of toys. This item is frequently easy to elicit in young children who are crawling in 4 point.

This item is scored using the generic scoring key (*i.e.* 1 = less than 10%, etc.).

*32. <u>Sitting on mat with feet in front: Attains 4 point over left side</u>

     0. does not initiate 4 point over left side
     1. initiates 4 point over left side
     2. partially attains 4 point over left side
     3. attains 4 point over left side

STARTING POSITION

Position the child on the mat in a sitting position with their legs comfortably in front of them. Note that this differs from item 30 (*i.e.* "W" sitting is not acceptable for this item).

INSTRUCTIONS

It is anticipated that children will move through some variation of left side sitting or move forward and to the left over their left leg. It is also expected that they will accomplish this by taking weight onto their arms. It is not important whether they take weight first onto one or both forearms and then extend their arms later or if they immediately take weight onto their hands. However, they may not assume prone first and then progress to 4 point from prone (assuming 4 point from prone is assessed in item 41).

Older children may respond to verbal instruction but many will require further explanation. Demonstration or "walking them through it" may be necessary.

Young children will again need to be enticed with strategic placement of toys. This item is frequently easy to elicit in young children who are crawling in 4 point.

This item is scored using the generic scoring key (*i.e.* 1 = less than 10%, etc.).

33. **Sitting on mat: Pivots 90°, without arms assisting**

     0. does not initiate pivoting
     1. initiates pivot
     2. pivots 90° with arms assisting
     3. pivots 90° without arms assisting

STARTING POSITION
The child may begin in any sitting position on the mat. The position of the arms will vary according to whether the arms are assisting or not. As well, the child must be reasonably stable in sitting to attempt this item.

INSTRUCTIONS
Instruct the child to pivot to the left or right (either direction is acceptable). Many children will benefit from demonstration. Younger children may pivot in pursuit of a toy. As with pivoting in prone, it is advisable to place the toy beyond 90° but still within their view. Unfortunately many young children will assume 4 point instead of pivoting.

For a score of 2, "arms assisting", the arms may assist in any manner (*i.e.* hands moving along the floor as well as the legs, or hands on the legs either for balance or to assist with moving them).

For a score of 3, "without arms assisting", the arms may not be perceived as helping to pivot in any manner. They may be positioned elsewhere on the body or in space (including clasped together).

*34. **Sitting on bench: Maintains, arms and feet free, 10 seconds**

     0. does not maintain sitting on bench
     1. maintains, arms propping and feet supported, 10 seconds
     2. maintains, arms free and feet supported, 10 seconds
     3. maintains, arms and feet free, 10 seconds

Position the child on the bench with knees at the edge and feet dangling. The position of the arms and support for the feet will depend on the ability of the child.

To test for a score of 3 the child must be on a large bench with feet dangling with no support (see Equipment section, p 43, for description of large bench). To test for a score of 1 or 2 the child may remain on the large bench and a small bench can be placed under the feet for support or the child can be placed on a small bench with feet on the floor (see Equipment section, p 43, for description of small bench).

INSTRUCTIONS
Place the child on the large bench as if a score of 3 was to be tested (*i.e.* feet dangling unsupported). If stable sitting is achieved ask the child to lift the arms to the "arms free" position. The therapist may let go of the child before or after the child assumes "arms free". Time the child for 10 seconds.

If the child is unable to maintain for 10 seconds, add support for the feet, then, if necessary, support the feet and allow the hand(s) to be propped.

Once it has been established at what level the child is to be tested, offer up to three trials at that level or up to three trials at more than one level (*i.e.* it is not necessary to count those trials as part of the three allowable trials when the therapist is trying to establish what the child will attempt). Remember that the child must maintain the position for 10 seconds to be credited at any level.

Note that any child who uses arm propping (regardless of whether or not the feet are free) does not meet the criterion for a score greater than 1.

*35. Standing: Attains sitting on small bench

    0. does not initiate sitting on small bench
    1. initiates sitting on small bench
    2. partially attains sitting on small bench
    3. attains sitting on small bench

STARTING POSITION
Position the child in standing in front of a small bench (see Equipment section, p 43, for description of small bench). It is acceptable to face toward or away from the bench or be parallel to it. The child may begin standing unsupported

or holding on to the bench with one or both hands, but leaning on the bench with any part of the trunk is not acceptable.

INSTRUCTIONS

This item is to demonstrate if children can lower themselves from standing to sitting on the bench. Children are expected to attain sitting on the bench using whatever manner they choose. Some may crawl onto the bench and turn around or they may lower themselves to sitting.

The older child should be instructed to sit on the bench. Younger children may respond better to demonstration or encouragement with toys. This item is scored using the generic scoring key (*i.e.* 1 = less than 10%, etc.). For children to obtain a score of 1 they must demonstrate some indication of trying to get onto the bench.

*36. <u>On the floor: Attains sitting on small bench</u>

    0. does not initiate sitting on small bench
    1. initiates sitting on small bench
    2. partially attains sitting on small bench
    3. attains sitting on small bench

STARTING POSITION

Position the child on the floor in front of the bench. "On the floor" is intended to be any position other than standing. This may include any lying or sitting position as well as variations of 4 point or kneeling. The child may face toward or away from the bench or be parallel to it.

INSTRUCTIONS

Contrary to item 35, this item is to demonstrate if children can raise themselves from the floor to sitting on a small bench. As in item 35 children may attain sitting on the small bench using whatever manner they choose. Many will assume standing first but some will attempt to pull themselves onto the bench without using standing in the process.

Ask older children to sit on the bench. Provide a demonstration if appropriate. Many children will need encouragement if this task requires a lot of effort physically. Strategic placement of toys may also help. This item is also scored using the generic scoring key (*i.e.* 1 = less than 10%, etc.). As with item 35 any child who demonstrates an attempt to get on the bench should receive a score of 1. This should include any children who attempt to raise themselves from their start position and are moving toward the bench. A score of 2 (10% to less than 100%) should be given to any children who are able to raise themselves to standing at the bench (or almost to standing using the bench for support).

Some therapists have expressed concerns with the generic scoring for this item. Remembering the start position and what is required to obtain a score of 3 should assist with calculating what percentage of the task the child has completed.

*37. On the floor: Attains sitting on large bench

> 0. does not initiate sitting on large bench
> 1. initiates sitting on large bench
> 2. partially attains sitting on large bench
> 3. attains sitting on large bench

STARTING POSITION

Position the child on the floor in front of the bench. "On the floor" is intended to be any position other than standing. This may include lying or sitting, or variations of 4 point or kneeling. (See Equipment section, p 43, for description of large bench.)

INSTRUCTIONS

This item is intended to determine if children can raise themselves from the floor to sitting on a large bench. As in items 35 and 36 children may use whatever method they choose.

Ask older children to climb onto the bench and assume any sitting position. Demonstration may be necessary for suggesting appropriate strategies. A lot of encouragement may be necessary to entice them to make the effort. Younger children often enjoy climbing onto tall furniture but may need further demonstration and encouragement to have them assume sitting.

This item is also scored using the generic scoring key (*i.e.* 1 = less than 10%, etc.). As with items 35 and 36, any child who demonstrates an attempt to get on the bench should receive a score of 1. This should include any children who attempt to raise themselves from their start position and are moving toward the bench. A score of 2 (10% to less than 100%) should be given to any children who are able to raise themselves to standing at the bench (or almost standing using the bench for support).

CRAWLING & KNEELING

This dimension includes 14 items that deal with various aspects of 4 point and high kneeling. These include the child's ability to:
• assume and/or maintain variations of 4 point and high kneeling
• move forward in prone, 4 point or high kneeling
• perform specific tasks in 4 point.
   The following terms employed in this dimension are defined in the Explanation of Terms at the end of this chapter (pp 124–129) and/or in the item(s) in which they occur as part of the instructions. They are listed in the order in which they appear:
• creep
• 4 point
• crawl
• hitch
• crawl reciprocally
• high kneeling
• holding on
• using arms
• arms free
• half kneeling
• kneel walk.

38. Prone: Creeps forward 1.8 m (6 ft)

   0. does not initiate creeping forward
   1. creeps forward <60 cm (2 ft)
   2. creeps forward 60 cm–1.5 m (2–5 ft)
   3. creeps forward 1.8 m (6 ft)

STARTING POSITION
Position the child comfortably in prone at one end of a 2.5 m (8 ft) mat.

Instruct the child to move forward on her/his stomach using arms and legs.

"Creeping" is defined as moving forward in prone, using the extremities, with the abdomen on the weight-bearing surface. This includes any variation of commando crawling.

Place a toy on the mat to provide a target for the child to creep toward. The toy should be placed beyond 1.8 m to avoid having the child creep less than 1.8 m and then reach for it. Use some part of the child's body (rather than the hand) to judge the distance moved. Younger children who can crawl in 4 point frequently do not understand this item even with demonstration. Setting up a low tunnel that does not allow crawling in 4 point may be helpful.

Another useful strategy to which the 4- to 8-year-old group responds very well is to have a "snake race", complete with hissing!

*39. 4 Point: Maintains, weight on hands and knees, 10 seconds

     0. does not maintain weight on hands and knees
     1. maintains weight on hands and knees, <3 seconds
     2. maintains weight on hands and knees, 3–9 seconds
     3. maintains weight on hands and knees, 10 seconds

STARTING POSITION
Position the child on the mat comfortably in 4 point; "4 point" is defined as weight-bearing on the hands and knees. The head, trunk and pelvis must be off the mat and/or the lower legs. Alignment, particularly of the arms and legs, may vary within the above limitations.

INSTRUCTIONS
Once children appear comfortable in the 4 point position, instruct them to maintain the position for the required time. Providing something to look at to hold their attention may help to accomplish this item. Therapists must remove their hands from the child before beginning to time the number of seconds. Any observable attempt to maintain the position once therapists remove their hands should be given a score of 1 (even if it is only momentary).

*40. 4 Point: Attains sitting, arms free

   0. does not initiate sitting
   1. initiates sitting
   2. attains sitting, arm(s) propping
   3. attains sitting, arms free

STARTING POSITION
Place the child on the mat comfortably in the 4 point position (the child must be able to maintain 4 point to attempt this item).

INSTRUCTIONS
Instruct the child to assume sitting. Younger children may require demonstration or need to be physically helped through the transition before attempting it themselves. The achievement of sitting, arms free, may require engaging them in hand games. For a score of 2 there may be one or two arms propping.

*41. Prone: Attains 4 point, weight on hands and knees

   0. does not initiate 4 point
   1. initiates 4 point
   2. partially attains 4 point
   3. attains 4 point, weight on hands and knees

STARTING POSITION
Position the child on the mat comfortably in prone.

INSTRUCTIONS
Instruct the child to assume 4 point. Remember that alignment in 4 point may vary, so long as the weight is on the hands and knees, and the head, trunk and pelvis, and/or the lower legs, are off the mat.

  Younger children will frequently assume 4 point spontaneously, but others may need to be encouraged verbally or with strategic placement of toys.

  This item is scored using the generic scoring key (*i.e.* 1 = less than 10%, etc.) to allow for the variations in initiating 4 point.

*42. <u>4 Point: Reaches forward with right arm, hand above shoulder level</u>

    0. does not initiate reaching forward with right arm
    1. initiates reaching forward with right arm
    2. partially reaches forward with right arm
    3. reaches forward with right arm, hand above shoulder level

STARTING POSITION

Position the child comfortably in 4 point on the mat. The child must be able
to maintain 4 point to attempt this item.

INSTRUCTIONS

Older children may simply be asked to reach forward with their right hand
above shoulder level. Many children will need to be encouraged to reach forward toward the therapist's hand or a toy. Placement of the toy is important
as it will be the cue that guides the child to extend the right arm forward and
reach above shoulder level. Alignment of the legs and left arm is not important,
so long as the criteria for 4 point continue to be maintained.

    This item is scored using the generic scoring key (*i.e.* 1 = less than 10%, etc.).

    The child who reaches forward and above shoulder level but lacks full elbow
extension (even though the hand is above shoulder level) should receive a score
of 3 for this item (reaching forward and above shoulder level is more important
than full elbow extension). However, the child must reach forward far enough
that the right hand has moved forward beyond the head.

*43. <u>4 Point: Reaches forward with left arm, hand above shoulder level</u>

    0. does not initiate reaching forward with left arm
    1. initiates reaching forward with left arm
    2. partially reaches forward with left arm
    3. reaches forward with left arm, hand above shoulder level

STARTING POSITION

Position the child comfortably in 4 point on the mat. The child must be able
to maintain 4 point to attempt this item.

INSTRUCTIONS

Older children may simply be asked to reach forward with their left hand above shoulder level. Many children will need to be encouraged to reach forward toward the therapist's hand or a toy. Placement of the toy is important as it will be the cue that guides the child to extend the left arm forward and reach above shoulder level. Alignment of the legs and right arm is not important, so long as the criteria for 4 point continue to be maintained.

This item is scored using the generic scoring key (*i.e.* 1 = less than 10%, etc.).

The child who reaches forward and above shoulder level but lacks full elbow extension (even though the hand is above shoulder level) should receive a score of 3 for this item (reaching forward and above shoulder level is more important than full elbow extension). However, the child must reach forward far enough that the left hand has moved forward beyond the head.

*44. 4 Point: Crawls or hitches forward 1.8 m (6 ft)

    0. does not initiate crawling or hitching forward
    1. crawls or hitches forward <60 cm (2 ft)
    2. crawls or hitches forward 60 cm–1.5 m (2–5 ft)
    3. crawls or hitches forward 1.8 m (6 ft)

STARTING POSITION
Position the child comfortably in 4 point at one end of a 2.5 m (8 ft) mat. The child must be able to maintain 4 point at least momentarily to attempt this item.

INSTRUCTIONS
Instruct the child to crawl forward or hitch to the end of the mat. "Crawling" is defined as moving on hands and knees. The arms and legs do not have to move alternately. "Hitching" is defined as moving jerkily. This may include "bunny hopping" or "bottom hitching" where the child moves forward using arms and/or legs while maintaining some variation of sitting. Note that the start position is 4 point even if the child is going to be using bottom hitching.

Placing a toy on the mat may be appropriate to provide a target for the child to crawl or hitch toward. The toy should be placed beyond 1.8 m to avoid having the child crawl less than 1.8 m and then reach for it. The therapist may also start with the toy close to the child and keep moving it gradually to entice the child to keep moving forward.

*45. **4 Point: Crawls reciprocally forward 1.8 m (6 ft)**

> 0. does not initiate crawling forward reciprocally
> 1. crawls reciprocally forward <60 cm (2 ft)
> 2. crawls reciprocally forward 60 cm–1.5 m (2–5 ft)
> 3. crawls reciprocally forward 1.8 m (6 ft)

STARTING POSITION
Position the child comfortably in 4 point at one end of a 2.5 m (8 ft) mat. The child must be able to maintain 4 point to attempt this item.

INSTRUCTIONS
Instruct the child to crawl forward reciprocally to the end of the mat. "Crawling reciprocally" is defined as moving on hands and knees with alternating movements of both the arms and the legs. These alternating movements do not necessarily need to be coordinated. Bunny hopping and bottom hitching are not acceptable.

Many children will need to be reminded to use reciprocal crawling (as opposed to bunny hopping). Placing a toy on the mat may be appropriate to provide a target for the child to crawl toward. The toy should be placed beyond 1.8 m to avoid having the child crawl less than 1.8 m and then reach for it. The therapist may also start with the toy close to the child and keep moving it gradually to entice the child to keep moving forward.

*46. **4 Point: Crawls up four steps on hands and knees/feet**

> 0. does not initiate crawling up steps
> 1. crawls up one step on hands and knees/feet
> 2. crawls up two or three steps on hands and knees/feet
> 3. crawls up four steps on hands and knees/feet

STARTING POSITION
Position the child comfortably in 4 point on the floor in front of a set of a minimum of four to six steps that are standard sized, *i.e.* approximately 18 cm (7 in) rise. If children prefer, they may begin in standing.

INSTRUCTIONS
Instruct the child to crawl up the steps. A young child may require demonstration

or further prompting with the use of toys. The therapist should be behind the child to reduce the possibility of injury from falling. Any variation of creeping or crawling is acceptable for this item, so long as the child is moving forward up the steps, one step at a time (*i.e.* moving up the steps backwards in sitting is not acceptable).

Both arms and legs must reach the fourth step to achieve a score of 3. Some children will stop when their hands reach the fourth step; the use of a set of six steps could ensure that both arms and legs will reach the required distance.

47. **4 Point: Crawls backwards down four steps on hands and knees/feet**

      0. does not initiate crawling backwards down steps
      1. crawls backwards down one step on hands and knees/feet
      2. crawls backwards down two or three steps on hands and knees/feet
      3. crawls backwards down four steps on hands and knees/feet

STARTING POSITION
Position the child comfortably in 4 point at the top of a minimum of four to six steps that are standard sized, *i.e.* approximately 18 cm (7 in) rise.

INSTRUCTIONS
Instruct the child to crawl down the steps one at a time. A young child may require demonstration or further prompting with the use of toys. The therapist should be behind the child to reduce the possibility of injury from falling. Many children are nervous attempting this activity and require close attention and encouragement. Be careful not to touch them when offering encouragement.

Any variation of creeping or crawling is acceptable for this item, so long as the child is moving backward feet first down the steps one step at a time (*i.e.* moving forwards in sitting or "sliding" down in prone is not acceptable).

Both arms and legs must reach the fourth step to achieve a score of 3. Many children will stop when their feet touch the floor. If a set of four steps has been used they have not met the criteria for both arms and legs moving the required distance.

INSTRUCTIONS

Instruct children to walk forward on their knees at least 10 steps. One step forward includes the movement of one leg from "push off" to floor contact. Note that for each of the three possible scores, 10 steps forward must be taken.

Several "test trials" may be needed to determine whether or not the child needs to be holding on to equipment, whether or not one or two hands will be used, and, if necessary, which equipment is best for the child to hold on to. It may also be necessary to test what surface is best for the child to kneel walk on, and whether the equipment will move forward easily.

STANDING

This dimension includes 13 items that deal with various aspects of standing. These include the child's ability to:
- maintain various standing positions
- assume standing from various positions
- perform specific tasks from the standing position.

Remember that all items including these are to be done with shoes removed.

The following terms employed in this dimension are defined in the Explanation of Terms at the end of this chapter (pp 124–129) and/or in the item(s) in which they occur as part of the instructions. They are listed in the order in which they appear:
- on the floor
- standing
- holding on
- arms free
- high kneeling
- half kneeling
- crashes
- using arms
- with control
- squat.

*52. On the floor: Pulls to stand at large bench

    0. does not initiate pulling to stand
    1. initiates pulling to stand
    2. partially pulls to stand
    3. pulls to stand at large bench

STARTING POSITION
Position the child on the floor in front of the bench. "On the floor" is intended to be any position other than standing. This may include any lying or sitting position as well as any variation of 4 point or kneeling. The child may be in any direction relative to the bench. Starting on the mat is also acceptable. (See Equipment section, p 43, for description of large bench.)

INSTRUCTIONS
Instruct the child to pull to stand at the bench.

Younger children may require demonstration or encouragement either verbally or with strategic placement of toys. The intent of this item is to determine the child's ability to pull to stand, not the quality of stand at completion.

This item is scored using the generic scoring key (*i.e.* 1 = less than 10%, etc.) to allow for the variations in pulling to stand and for the variations in starting position.

To obtain a score of 3, children must be on their feet in the upright position, but they may be leaning on the tall bench with any part of their body and/or their arms.

*53. Standing: Maintains, arms free, 3 seconds

    0. does not maintain standing, holding on
    1. maintains, two hands holding on, 3 seconds
    2. maintains, one hand holding on, 3 seconds
    3. maintains, arms free, 3 seconds

STARTING POSITION
Position the child comfortably in the standing position, preferably on the floor (as opposed to the mat).

"Standing" is defined as being in the upright position on the feet. Alignment, particularly of the trunk and lower extremities, may vary. The standing position will also vary, depending on whether or not the child is holding on and whether it is with one or two hands. (Review "holding on" in the Explanation of Terms, p 128.)

To obtain a score of 3 the child may be positioned standing on the floor with or without support in preparation for letting go and standing, arms free. (Review "arms free" in the Explanation of Terms, p 128.) To obtain a score of 2 or 1 the child must be positioned holding on to any of the listed equipment with one or two hands.

INSTRUCTIONS

This item may require a few "test trials" to determine whether the child will be "holding on" and whether one or two hands will be used. Once this has been determined, the three trials for scoring can then begin.

To obtain a score of 3, instruct the child to let go of any support and stand, arms free, for 3 seconds.

To obtain a score of 2, instruct the child to stand, holding on to the equipment with one hand, for 3 seconds. Leaning on the equipment with any part of the body other than the one hand is not acceptable.

To obtain a score of 1, instruct the child to stand, holding on to the equipment with two hands, for 3 seconds. Leaning on the forearms or touching the equipment with other parts of the body is acceptable provided that the weight is being taken through the arms and legs (rather than the trunk).

*54. <u>Standing: Holding on to large bench with one hand, lifts right foot, 3 seconds</u>

    0. does not initiate lifting right foot
    1. holding on to large bench with two hands, lifts right foot, <3 seconds
    2. holding on to large bench with two hands, lifts right foot, 3 seconds
    3. holding on to large bench with one hand, lifts right foot, 3 seconds

STARTING POSITION

Position the child comfortably in the standing position, preferably on the floor (as opposed to the mat), holding on to the large bench. Facing the bench is preferable, although the child may also be positioned with the bench at the side, especially for a score of 3.

To obtain a score of 3, the child begins holding on to the bench with one hand.

To obtain a score of 1 or 2, the child begins holding on to the bench with two hands.

The child may not lean on the bench with the trunk, but leaning on one or both forearms is acceptable depending on whether a score of 3 (one hand) or 1 or 2 (two hands) is being attempted.

INSTRUCTIONS

This item may require a few "test trials" to determine whether the child will begin holding on to the bench with one or two hands. The leg lifted must clear the floor completely.

To obtain a score of 3, instruct the child to lift the right leg for 3 seconds while holding on with one hand. It is not acceptable to lift the right leg while holding on with two hands and then let go with one hand.

To obtain a score of 1 or 2, instruct the child to lift the right leg while holding on with both hands. Time the action to determine whether the 3 second requirement is achieved.

Younger children may be enticed to lift either leg by preparing to step on a toy or putting on their pants, etc.

*55. <u>Standing: Holding on to large bench with one hand, lifts left foot, 3 seconds</u>

    0. does not initiate lifting left foot
    1. holding on to large bench with two hands, lifts left foot, <3 seconds
    2. holding on to large bench with two hands, lifts left foot, 3 seconds
    3. holding on to large bench with one hand, lifts left foot, 3 seconds

STARTING POSITION

Position the child comfortably in the standing position, preferably on the floor (rather than the mat) holding on to the large bench. Facing the bench is preferable, although the child may also be positioned with the bench at the side, especially for a score of 3.

To obtain a score of 3, the child begins holding on to the bench with one hand.

To obtain a score of 1 or 2 the child begins holding on to the bench with two hands.

The child may not lean on the bench with the trunk, but leaning on one or both forearms is acceptable depending on whether a score of 3 (one hand) or 1 or 2 (two hands) is being attempted.

INSTRUCTIONS

This item may require a few "test trials" to determine whether the child will begin holding on to the bench with one or two hands. The leg lifted must clear the floor completely.

To obtain a score of 3, instruct the child to lift the left leg for 3 seconds while holding on with one hand. It is not acceptable to lift the left leg while holding on with two hands and then let go with one hand.

To obtain a score of 1 or 2, instruct the child to lift the left leg while holding on with both hands. Time the action to determine whether the 3 second requirement is achieved.

Younger children may be enticed to lift either leg by preparing to step on a toy or putting on their pants, etc.

*56. <u>Standing: Maintains, arms free, 20 seconds</u>

    0. does not maintain standing, arms free
    1. maintains, arms free <3 seconds
    2. maintains, arms free 3–19 seconds
    3. maintains, arms free 20 seconds

STARTING POSITION

Position the child comfortably in the standing position preferably on the floor (rather than the mat). The child may begin with or without support in preparation for letting go and standing, arms free. (Review "standing" and "arms free" in the Explanation of Terms, pp 125–6, 128.)

INSTRUCTIONS

This item differs from item 53 in that it is the time that varies rather than the support. Children may adjust their stance but may not take a step in any direction. Older children may be encouraged to help "count the seconds". Younger children may need to be engaged in hand games, etc., to encourage them to remain standing rather than walking.

*57. **Standing: Lifts left foot, arms free, 10 seconds**

> 0. does not lift left foot, arms free
> 1. lifts left foot, arms free, <3 seconds
> 2. lifts left foot, arms free, 3–9 seconds
> 3. lifts left foot, arms free, 10 seconds

STARTING POSITION
Position the child comfortably in standing, arms free. S/he should be standing on the floor. The mat may be used to reduce the possibility of injury from falling, although it may make this item more difficult. (Review "standing" and "arms free" in the Explanation of Terms, pp 125–6, 128.)

INSTRUCTIONS
Instruct the child to lift the left foot so that it is clear of the floor and maintain standing on the right leg for up to 10 seconds.

Older children can be encouraged to maintain the position as long as possible by making them aware of the timing process. Younger children may require demonstration (either visual or "hands on") to ensure that they understand this item, and then further encouragement may be required to maintain the position as long as possible.

*58. **Standing: Lifts right foot, arms free, 10 seconds**

> 0. does not lift right foot, arms free
> 1. lifts right foot, arms free, <3 seconds
> 2. lifts right foot, arms free, 3–9 seconds
> 3. lifts right foot, arms free, 10 seconds

STARTING POSITION
Position the child comfortably in standing, arms free. S/he should be standing

on the floor. The mat may be used to reduce the possibility of injury from falling, although it may make this item more difficult. (Review "standing" and "arms free" in the Explanation of Terms, pp 125–6, 128.)

INSTRUCTIONS
Instruct the child to lift the right foot so that it is clear of the floor, and maintain standing on the left leg for up to 10 seconds.

Older children can be encouraged to maintain the position as long as possible by making them aware of the timing process. Younger children may require demonstration (either visual or "hands on") to ensure that they understand this item, and then further encouragement may be required to maintain the position as long as possible.

*59. Sitting on small bench: Attains standing without using arms

    0. does not initiate standing
    1. initiates standing
    2. attains standing using arms
    3. attains standing without using arms

STARTING POSITION
Position the child sitting on the small bench. If the small bench is the appropriate height, the child will be sitting with feet flat on the floor and knees flexed at 90°.

INSTRUCTIONS
Instruct the child to stand up. Younger children may need an incentive such as a toy in front of them on a table or in the therapist's hand to encourage them to stand rather than getting down on the floor.

To obtain a score of 3, children must achieve standing, arms free, without any assistance from their arms on the bench or their body in the transition.

To obtain a score of 2, children can achieve standing, arms free, by using their arms on the bench or their body to help them in the transition from sitting to standing.

To obtain a score of 1, the children must initiate an attempt at standing from the bench.

*60. <u>High kneeling: Attains standing through half kneeling on right knee,</u> <u>without using arms</u>

   0. does not initiate standing
   1. initiates standing
   2. attains standing using arm (s)
   3. attains standing through half kneeling on right knee, without using arms

STARTING POSITION
Position the child comfortably on the mat in high kneeling, arms free. (Review "high kneeling" and "arms free" in the Explanation of Terms, pp 125, 128.)

INSTRUCTIONS
Instruct the child to assume standing from high kneeling without using any external support such as furniture or the floor. Demonstration may be necessary. This item may require several "test trials" to determine whether the child will be using arm(s) and whether half kneeling will be used in the transition from high kneeling to stand.

   To obtain a score of 3, standing must be assumed from high kneeling without any assistance from the child's arms either on the mat or the body. Half kneeling on the right knee must be used in the transition from high kneeling to stand. (Review "half kneeling" in the Explanation of Terms, p 125.)

   To obtain a score of 2, standing must be assumed from high kneeling. In this instance, the child's arms may assist either on the mat or the body. Although half kneeling on the right knee may be used in transition, it is not necessary. Other positions such as squatting on hands and feet are also acceptable.

   To obtain a score of 1, the child must demonstrate an attempt to assume standing from high kneeling.

*61. <u>High kneeling: Attains standing through half kneeling on left knee,</u> <u>without using arms</u>

   0. does not initiate standing
   1. initiates standing
   2. attains standing using arm (s)
   3. attains standing through half kneeling on left knee, without using arms

STARTING POSITION
Position the child comfortably on the mat in high kneeling, arms free. (Review "high kneeling" and "arms free" in the Explanation of Terms, pp 125, 128.)

INSTRUCTIONS
Instruct the child to assume standing from high kneeling without using any external support such as furniture or the floor. Demonstration may be necessary. This item may require several "test trials" to determine whether the child will be using arm(s) and whether half kneeling will be used in the transition from high kneeling to stand.

To obtain a score of 3, standing must be assumed from high kneeling without any assistance from the child's arms either on the mat or the body. Half kneeling on the left knee must be used in the transition from high kneeling to stand. (Review "half kneeling" in the Explanation of Terms, p 125.)

To obtain a score of 2, standing must be assumed from high kneeling. In this instance, the child's arms may assist either on the mat or the body. Although half kneeling on the left knee may be used in transition, it is not necessary. Other positions such as squatting on hands and feet are also acceptable.

To obtain a score of 1, the child must demonstrate an attempt to assume standing from high kneeling.

*62. <u>Standing: Lowers to sitting on floor with control, arms free</u>

    0. does not lower to floor
    1. lowers to sitting on floor, but "crashes" down
    2. lowers to sitting on floor with control, using arm(s) or holding on
    3. lowers to sitting on floor with control, arms free

STARTING POSITION
Position the child comfortably in standing on the floor or mat. The child must be able to stand, arms free, to attempt this item, although to obtain a score of 1 or 2, holding on to any equipment is acceptable once lowering to sitting has been initiated.

INSTRUCTIONS
Instruct the child to lower to sitting on the floor. This may include any sitting position. Several "test trials" may be required to determine whether the arms

will be used or equipment is required for "holding on". Testing may then begin.

To obtain a score of 3, the child must lower to sitting on the floor with control without using the arms on the floor or the body for assistance. "With control" implies that the movement is regulated or directed.

To obtain a score of 2, the child must lower to sitting on the floor with control, but the arms may be used for balance or support on the floor or the body, or the child may hold on to any of the listed equipment (or a suitable substitute).

To obtain a score of 1, the child must lower to sitting on the floor, but it does not have to be controlled (*i.e.* crashing). "Crash" is defined as "to fall, collide or collapse", but there must be obvious intent (as opposed to accidentally falling to the floor).

*63. Standing: Attains squat, arms free

    0. does not initiate squat
    1. initiates squat
    2. attains squat, using arm(s) or holding on
    3. attains squat, arms free

STARTING POSITION
Position the child comfortably in standing on the floor or mat. The child must be able to stand, arms free, to attempt this item, although to obtain a score of 1 or 2, holding on to any equipment is acceptable once squatting has been initiated.

INSTRUCTIONS
Instruct the child to lower to the squat position. "Squat" is defined as "crouching close to the ground" or "sitting on the heels with knees bent". For the purposes of this measure, both the hips/waist and knees must be flexed to greater than 90°. Several "test trials" may be required to determine whether the arms will be used or whether equipment is required for "holding on". Testing may then begin.

To obtain a score of 3, the child must attain the squat position, arms free. (Review "arms free" in Explanation of Terms, p 128.)

To obtain a score of 2, the child must also attain the squat position but the arms may be used on the body or floor for balance or support, or the child may hold on to any of the listed equipment (or a suitable substitute).

To obtain a score of 1, the child must initiate squat using any of the above strategies.

*64. Standing: Picks up object from floor, arms free, returns to standing

      0. does not initiate picking up object from floor
      1. initiates picking up object from floor
      2. picks up object from floor, using arm(s) or holding on
      3. picks up object from floor, arms free, returns to standing

STARTING POSITION

Position the child comfortably in standing on the floor or mat. The child must be able to stand, arms free, to attempt this item, although to obtain a score of 1 or 2, holding on to any equipment once they initiate picking up the object.

Place a small toy on the floor in front of the child.

INSTRUCTIONS

Instruct the child to pick up the toy and regain standing. Several "test trials" may be required to determine whether the arm(s) will be used or whether equipment is required for "holding on". Then testing may begin.

To obtain a score of 3, the child must pick up the toy from the floor and regain standing without using the arm(s) for support or balance on the floor, the body or any equipment.

To obtain a score of 2, the child must also pick up the toy from the floor and regain standing but the arm(s) may be used for support or balance on the body or floor, or the child may hold on to any of the listed equipment (or a substitute).

To obtain a score of 1, the child must initiate picking up the toy from the floor using any of the above strategies.

WALKING, RUNNING & JUMPING

This dimension includes 24 items that deal with a variety of activities that begin in standing. These include the child's ability to:
• engage in a variety of walking activities
• perform specific tasks such as walking up and down stairs or kicking a ball
• engage in a variety of jumping activities.

Remember that all items, including the above, are to be performed with shoes removed.

Where the starting position is described simply as "standing" without any other descriptions, it is implied that the child begins standing, arms free. This includes not holding on with hands as well as not leaning on furniture, etc. (even though they may be "hands free"). This applies to items 69–83 and 86–88.

Where the activity is described simply as "walks", "jumps", etc., and the starting position is simply "standing", it is also implied that the child performs the activity arms free (*i.e.* without any support either through the arms or by leaning). This also applies to items 69–83 and 86–88.

The following terms employed in this dimension are defined in the Explanation of Terms at the end of this chapter (pp 124–129) and/or in the item(s) in which they occur as part of the instructions. They are listed in the order in which they appear.
• cruise one step
• walk forward one step
• walk backward one step
• arms free
• consecutive steps
• run
• walk quickly
• kick
• jump
• both feet simultaneously
• stand on one foot
• hop
• walks up/down one step.

*65. Standing, two hands on large bench: Cruises five steps to right

    0. does not initiate cruising to right
    1. initiates cruising, <1 complete step to right
    2. cruises 1–4 steps to right
    3. cruises 5 steps to right

STARTING POSITION
Position the child in standing facing the large bench and holding on with two hands (see description of large bench under Equipment, p 43). Leaning on forearms or touching the equipment with other parts of the body is acceptable provided that the weight is being taken through the arms and legs (as opposed to the trunk). The child should be at one end of the bench, and the bench should be long enough to allow five steps to the right (parallel bars may be substituted).

INSTRUCTIONS
Instruct the child to walk sideways (cruise) up to five steps to the right. Demonstration (including "hands on") may be required to help the child understand the request. Placing an incentive such as a favourite toy on the bench to the right of the child may elicit the desired response. Movement sideways of both legs (one at a time) constitutes one step in cruising.

    The child may turn slightly to cruise but must still be stepping sideways (as opposed to walking forward).

*66. Standing, two hands on large bench: Cruises five steps to left

    0. does not initiate cruising to left
    1. initiates cruising, <1 complete step to left
    2. cruises 1–4 steps to left
    3. cruises 5 steps to left

STARTING POSITION
Position the child in standing facing the large bench, and holding on with two hands (see description of large bench under Equipment, p 43). Leaning on forearms or touching the equipment with other parts of the body is acceptable provided that the weight is being taken through the arms and legs (as opposed

to the trunk). The child should be at one end of the bench and the bench should be long enough to allow five steps to the left (parallel bars may be substituted).

INSTRUCTIONS
Instruct the child to walk sideways (cruise) up to five steps to the left. Demonstration (including "hands on") may be required to help the child understand the request. Placing an incentive such as a favourite toy on the bench to the left of the child may elicit the desired response. Movement sideways of both legs (one at a time) constitutes one step in cruising.

The child may turn slightly to cruise but must still be stepping sideways (as opposed to walking forward).

*67. <u>Standing, two hands held: Walks forward 10 steps</u>

    0. does not initiate walking forward
    1. walks forward <3 steps
    2. walks forward 3–9 steps
    3. walks forward 10 steps

STARTING POSITION
Position the child in standing with both hands held by the therapist. (Review "standing" in the Explanation of Terms, p 125–6.) The therapist should be in front of the child, if possible, to reduce the inclination to facilitate walking. By holding the child's hands the therapist can provide support or balance, but the child must take most of the weight through the legs to maintain upright.

INSTRUCTIONS
Instruct the child to walk forward with two hands held, as far as possible, up to 10 steps. One step forward includes the movement forward of one leg from push off to floor contact or heel strike. Verbal encouragement or a visible incentive to walk towards may provide additional motivation to walk further. The steps must be consecutive; there may be a short pause of 1 or 2 seconds during walking, but any longer should be considered the end of the trial.

*68. Standing, one hand held: Walks forward 10 steps

    0. does not initiate walking forward
    1. walks forward <3 steps
    2. walks forward 3–9 steps
    3. walks forward 10 steps

STARTING POSITION
Position the child in standing with one hand (either hand) held by the therapist. (Review "standing" in the Explanation of Terms, p 125–6.) The therapist may be in front of the child or to the side, but, as in item 67, the therapist should be providing support or balance while the child is taking most of the weight through the legs.

INSTRUCTIONS
Instruct the child to walk forward, with one hand held, as far as possible, up to 10 steps. One step forward includes the movement forward of one leg from push off to floor contact or heel strike. Verbal encouragement or a visible incentive to walk towards may provide additional motivation to walk further. As in item 67, the steps must be consecutive; there may be a short pause of 1 or 2 seconds during walking, but any longer should be considered the end of the trial.

*69. Standing: Walks forward 10 steps

    0. does not initiate walking forward
    1. walks forward <3 steps
    2. walks forward 3–9 steps
    3. walks forward 10 steps

STARTING POSITION
The child must be able to stand, arms free, to attempt this item. Position the child comfortably in standing on the floor. (Review "standing" and "arms free" in the Explanation of Terms, pp 125–6, 128.)

INSTRUCTIONS
Instruct the child to walk forward as far as possible up to 10 steps. One step forward includes the movement forward of one leg from push off to floor contact

or heel strike. Verbal encouragement or a visible incentive to walk towards may provide additional motivation to walk further. As in items 67 and 68, the steps must be consecutive; there may be a short pause of 1 or 2 seconds during walking, but any longer should be considered the end of the trial.

*70. Standing: Walks forward 10 steps, stops, turns 180°, returns

    0. walks forward 10 steps, does not stop without falling
    1. walks forward 10 steps, stops, does not initiate turn
    2. walks forward 10 steps, stops, turns <180°
    3. walks forward 10 steps, stops, turns 180°, returns

STARTING POSITION
The child must be able to stand, arms free, to attempt this item. Position the child comfortably in standing on the floor. (Review "standing" and "arms free" in the Explanation of Terms, pp 125–6, 128.)

INSTRUCTIONS
Instruct the child on the various requirements for this item. The child must be able to walk forward, arms free, to attempt this item. Several "test trials" may be required to ensure that all aspects are understood. Be careful to emphasize the correct sequencing. For example, the child must stop and then turn (as opposed to turning then stopping). It is acceptable for the therapist to provide cues during each trial so long as the child is not touched. For a score of 3, it is implied by the word "returns" that the child returns to the starting position, but it is not necessary to count the steps. The important aspects are whether the child can: walk forward and stop without falling; and walk forward and turn 180° and begin walking again.

*71. Standing: Walks backward 10 steps

    0. does not initiate walking backward
    1. walks backward <3 steps
    2. walks backward 3–9 steps
    3. walks backward 10 steps

STARTING POSITION
The child must be able to stand, arms free, to attempt this item. Position the

child comfortably in standing on the floor. (Review "standing" and "arms free" in the Explanation of Terms, pp 125–6, 128.)

INSTRUCTIONS
Instruct the child to walk backward, arms free as far as possible up to 10 steps. One step backward includes the movement backward of one leg (as in walking forward). The size of the step is not important so long as the child is moving backwards. The steps must be consecutive. There may be a short pause of 1 to 2 seconds during walking, but a longer interval should be considered the end of the trial. Verbal encouragement or guidance may assist with motivating the child to continue.

*72. Standing: Walks forward 10 steps, carrying a large object with two hands

    0. does not initiate walking, carrying large object
    1. walks forward 10 steps, carrying a small object with one hand
    2. walks forward 10 steps, carrying a small object with two hands
    3. walks forward 10 steps, carrying a large object with two hands

STARTING POSITION
The child must be able to stand, arms free, to attempt this item. Position the child comfortably in standing on the floor. (Review "standing" and "arms free" in the Explanation of Terms, pp 125–6, 128.)

INSTRUCTIONS
The child must be able to walk forward, arms free to attempt this item. Several "test trials" may be necessary to determine whether a large or small object will be used. A small object is considered one that is easily carried by the child with one or two hands (*e.g.* a small doll or truck). A large object is considered one that must be carried with two hands (*e.g.* a soccer ball or balloon).

Instruct the child to carry the object while walking forward, arms free. Note that 10 steps forward are required for each of the three scores, and the size of the object and number of hands are the variables.

Having younger children carry the object from one person to another may assist with achieving this item.

***73. <u>Standing: Walks forward 10 consecutive steps between parallel lines</u>
<u>20 cm (8 in) apart</u>**

> 0. does not initiate walking forward between parallel lines 20 cm (8 in)
>   apart
> 1. walks forward <3 consecutive steps between parallel lines 20 cm (8 in)
>   apart
> 2. walks forward 3–9 consecutive steps between parallel lines 20 cm
>   (8 in) apart
> 3. walks forward 10 consecutive steps between parallel lines 20 cm (8 in)
>   apart

STARTING POSITION
The child must be able to stand, arms free, to attempt this item. Position the
child comfortably on the floor at the beginning of two parallel lines, 20 cm
(8 in) apart and 6 m (20 ft) long. (Review "standing" and "arms free" in the
Explanation of Terms, pp 125–6, 128.)

INSTRUCTIONS
The child must be able to walk forward, arms free, to attempt this item. In
order to meet the criteria for walking between the lines, part of the foot may
touch the line but not go over it.

The steps must be consecutive (*i.e.* without interruption). As well as not
having pauses between steps greater than 2 seconds, the required number of
steps must be taken without going over the line. Once either foot goes over
the line, a new trial must begin.

Instruct the child to walk forward carefully keeping both feet between the
lines. Demonstration will be required for most children.

***74. <u>Standing: Walks forward 10 consecutive steps on a straight line</u>
<u>2 cm (w in) wide</u>**

> 0. does not initiate walking forward on a straight line 2 cm (w in) wide
> 1. walks forward <3 consecutive steps on a straight line 2 cm (w in)
>   wide
> 2. walks forward 3–9 consecutive steps on a straight line 2 cm (w in)
>   wide
> 3. walks forward 10 consecutive steps on a straight line 2 cm (w in) wide

STARTING POSITION

The child must be able to stand, arms free, to attempt this item. Position the child comfortably in standing on the floor at the beginning of a straight line 2 cm (w in) wide and 6 m (20 ft) long. (Review "standing" and "arms free" in the Explanation of Terms, pp 125–6, 128.)

INSTRUCTIONS

The child must be able to walk forward, arms free, to attempt this item. In order to meet the criteria for walking on the line, part of the foot must stay on the line. The steps must be consecutive. As well as not having pauses between steps greater than 2 seconds, the required number of steps must be taken with part of the foot staying on the line. Once either foot goes off the line, a new trial must begin.

Instruct the child to walk forward carefully, keeping both feet on the line. Demonstration will be required for most children.

*75. <u>Standing: Steps over stick at knee level, right foot leading</u>

      0. does not initiate stepping over stick, right foot leading
      1. steps over stick 5–7.5 cm (2–3 in) high, right foot leading
      2. steps over stick at mid-calf level, right foot leading
      3. steps over stick at knee level, right foot leading

STARTING POSITION

The child must be able to stand, arms free, to attempt this item. Position the child comfortably in standing on the floor. (Review "standing" and "arms free" in the Explanation of Terms, pp 125–6, 128.) The therapist should be in front of the child or to the side, holding the stick horizontally.

INSTRUCTIONS

The child must be able to walk forward, arms free, to attempt this item. Several "practice" trials may be necessary to determine at what height the stick should be held. It may be useful to begin at the lowest level and gradually raise it to the appropriate level. The testing may then begin.

Instruct the child to step over the stick leading with the right foot. Both legs must clear the stick at the specified level. The child must clear the stick, arms free, and finish without falling.

113

*76. <u>Standing: Steps over stick at knee level, left foot leading</u>

    0. does not initiate stepping over stick, left foot leading
    1. steps over stick 5–7.5 cm (2–3 in) high, left foot leading
    2. steps over stick at mid-calf level, left foot leading
    3. steps over stick at knee level, left foot leading

STARTING POSITION
The child must be able to stand, arms free, to attempt this item. Position the
child comfortably in standing on the floor. (Review "standing" and "arms free"
in the Explanation of Terms, pp 125–6, 128.) The therapist should be in front
of the child or to the side, holding the stick horizontally.

INSTRUCTIONS
The child must be able to walk forward, arms free, to attempt this item. Several
"practice" trials may be necessary to determine at what height the stick should
be held. It may be useful to begin at the lowest level and gradually raise it to
the appropriate level. The testing may then begin.
    Instruct the child to step over the stick leading with the left foot. Both legs
must clear the stick at the specified level. The child must clear the stick, arms
free, and finish without falling.

*77. <u>Standing: Runs 4.5 m (15 ft), stops and returns</u>

    0. does not initiate running
    1. initiates running by walking quickly
    2. runs <4.5 m (15 ft)
    3. runs 4.5 m (15 ft), stops and returns

STARTING POSITION
The child must be able to stand, arms free, to attempt this item. Position the
child comfortably in standing on the floor. (Review "standing" and "arms free"
in the Explanation of Terms, pp 125–6, 128.)

INSTRUCTIONS
The child must be able to walk forward, arms free, to attempt this item. Several
"test trials" may be necessary to determine if running or walking quickly will
be used. If running is a possibility, instruct the child to run to a destination

4.5 m (15 ft) away, stop and run back to the starting point. For the child to be classified as "running", there must be an instant where both feet are off the floor at the same time. In walking quickly both feet may be on the floor at the same time even though it is very brief. Many children will benefit from demonstration and some may benefit from the therapist performing the item at the same time.

For a score of 3, the child must run 4.5 m (15 ft), stop without falling, turn and run back to the starting point.

For a score of 2, the child must run up to 4.5 m (15 ft).

For a score of 1, the child must initiate running by walking quickly up to 4.5 m (15 ft).

Some children will achieve a level that does not fit any of these descriptions. In each case you must choose the lowest score that best describes the observed performance; for example, if the child runs 6 m (20 ft), stops and falls, a score of 2 should be awarded.

*78. <u>Standing: Kicks ball with right foot</u>

    0. does not initiate kicking
    1. lifts right foot, does not kick
    2. kicks ball with right foot, but falls
    3. kicks ball with right foot

STARTING POSITION
The child must be able to stand, arms free, to attempt this item. Position the child comfortably in standing on the floor. (Review "standing" and "arms free" in the Explanation of Terms, pp 125–6, 128.)

INSTRUCTIONS
Although it is likely that most children who attempt this item will be able to walk, arms free, it is not a prerequisite.

Place the ball on the floor in front of the child. The position of the ball is not critical as long as it is at least 10 cm (4 in) in front of the child's feet. Instruct the child to kick the ball with the right foot. To be considered a "kick" the right foot must clear the floor when the ball is contacted, and the ball must move from the impact of the foot.

For a score of 3, the child must kick the ball without falling. Momentarily losing one's balance or taking steps to maintain or recover balance is acceptable.

For any score, the right foot must clear the floor.

Many children have fun performing this item. The "accomplished kickers" often take an extra little step when performing this item and this should be considered acceptable. However, there are some less competent children who can only "kick" the ball by shuffling carefully forward and "colliding" with the ball to move it forward. These children must stand still and kick the ball as described. If they meet these criteria and include an extra little step as well this is also acceptable.

*79. Standing: Kicks ball with left foot

    0. does not initiate kicking
    1. lifts left foot, does not kick
    2. kicks ball with left foot, but falls
    3. kicks ball with left foot

STARTING POSITION
The child must be able to stand, arms free, to attempt this item. Position the child comfortably in standing on the floor. (Review "standing" and "arms free" in the Explanation of Terms, pp 125–6, 128.)

INSTRUCTIONS
Although it is likely that most children who attempt this item will be able to walk arms free, it is not a prerequisite.

Place the ball on the floor in front of the child. The position of the ball is not critical as long as it is at least 10 cm (4 in) in front of the child's feet. Instruct the child to kick the ball with the left foot. To be considered a "kick" the right foot must clear the floor when the ball is contacted, and the ball must move from the impact of the foot.

For a score of 3, the child must kick the ball without falling. Momentarily losing one's balance or taking steps to maintain or recover balance is acceptable.

For any score, the left foot must clear the floor.

Many children have fun performing this item. The "accomplished kickers" often take an extra little step when performing this item and this should be considered acceptable. However, there are some less competent children who can only "kick" the ball by shuffling carefully forward and "colliding" with the ball to move it forward. These children must stand still and kick the ball as described. If they meet these criteria and include an extra little step as well this is also acceptable.

*80. Standing: Jumps 30 cm (12 in) high, both feet simultaneously

    0. does not initiate jump
    1. jumps <5 cm (2 in) high, both feet simultaneously
    2. jumps 5–28 cm (2–11 in) high, both feet simultaneously
    3. jumps 30 cm (12 in) high, both feet simultaneously

STARTING POSITION
The child must be able to stand, arms free to attempt this item. Position the child comfortably in standing on the floor. (Review "standing" and "arms free" in the Explanation of Terms, pp 125–6, 128.)

INSTRUCTIONS
Although it is very likely that children who attempt this item will be able to walk, arms free, it is not a prerequisite. To be classified as a jump both feet must clear the floor. The child must jump and land, arms free, without falling, to receive credit for any score.

    Instruct the child to jump as high as s/he can, both feet simultaneously. The criterion for "both feet simultaneously" is that both feet are off the floor at the same time, even though both feet may not necessarily take off and land simultaneously. The height jumped is the distance that both feet clear off the ground.

*81. Standing: Jumps forward 30 cm (12 in), both feet simultaneously

    0. does not initiate jumping forward, both feet simultaneously
    1. jumps forward <5 cm (2 in), both feet simultaneously
    2. jumps forward 5–28 cm (2–11 in), both feet simultaneously
    3. jumps forward 30 cm (12 in), both feet simultaneously

STARTING POSITION
The child must be able to stand, arms free, to attempt this item. Position the

child comfortably in standing on the floor with the toes touching a visible line on the floor. (Review "standing" and "arms free" in the Explanation of Terms, pp 125–6, 128.)

Place two parallel lines 30 cm (12 in) apart on the floor that can be easily seen by the child.

INSTRUCTIONS
The child must jump and land, arms free, without falling to receive credit for any score. To be classified as a jump both feet must clear the floor.

Instruct the child to jump as far forward as s/he can, both feet simultaneously. (Review "both feet simultaneously" in Explanation of Terms, p 127.) The distance jumped is the distance cleared by *both* feet.

*82. **Standing: Hops on right foot 10 times within a 60 cm (24 in) circle**

    0. does not initiate hopping on right foot
    1. hops on right foot <3 times within a 60 cm (24 in) circle
    2. hops on right foot 3–9 times within a 60 cm (24 in) circle
    3. hops on right foot 10 times within a 60 cm (24 in) circle

STARTING POSITION
The child must be able to stand, arms free, to attempt this item. Position the child comfortably in standing, arms free, and within a clearly marked circle, 60 cm (24 in) in diameter.

INSTRUCTIONS
Instruct the child to hop as many times as possible (up to 10 times) while staying within the circle (*i.e.* part of the right foot must stay in the circle). If the child "travels" within the circle but consistently stays within a 60 cm (24 in) diameter it is acceptable to allow a "strategic" starting position within the circle. For example, if the child consistently tends to travel forward slightly it is acceptable to start at the edge of the circle.

To be classified as a "hop" the left foot must not touch the floor at any time, and the right foot must clear the floor and land without the child falling. The hopping must be done arms free. (Review "arms free" in the Explanation of Terms, p 128.)

The hops must be consecutive. As well as not having pauses between hops greater than 2 seconds, the required number of hops must be taken without going out of the circle, touching the floor with the left foot, touching anything for support or balance with the hand(s), or falling. Once any of these interruptions occur, a new trial must begin.

*83. Standing: Hops on left foot 10 times within a 60 cm (24 in) circle

    0. does not initiate hopping on left foot
    1. hops on left foot <3 times within a 60 cm (24 in) circle
    2. hops on left foot 3–9 times within a 60 cm (24 in) circle
    3. hops on left foot 10 times within a 60 cm (24 in) circle

STARTING POSITION
The child must be able to stand, arms free, to attempt this item. Position the child comfortably in standing, arms free, and within a clearly marked circle, 60 cm (24 in) in diameter.

INSTRUCTIONS
Instruct the child to hop as many times as possible (up to 10 times) while staying within the circle (*i.e.* part of the left foot must stay in the circle). If the child "travels" within the circle but consistently stays within a 60 cm (24 in) diameter it is acceptable to allow a "strategic" starting position within the circle. For example, if the child consistently tends to travel forward slightly it is acceptable to start at the edge of the circle.

    To be classified as a "hop" the right foot must not touch the floor at any time, and the left foot must clear the floor and land without the child falling. The hopping must be done arms free. (Review "arms free" in the Explanation of Terms, p 128.)

    The hops must be consecutive. As well as not having pauses between hops greater than 2 seconds, the required number of hops must be taken without going out of the circle, touching the floor with the right foot, touching anything for support or balance with the hand(s), or falling. Once any of these interruptions occur, a new trial must begin.

*84. Standing, holding one rail: Walks up four steps, holding one rail, alternating feet

    0. does not initiate walking up steps, holding rail
    1. walks up 2 steps, holding rail, same foot leads consistently
    2. walks up 4 steps, holding rail, alternating feet inconsistently
    3. walks up 4 steps, holding rail, alternating feet

STARTING POSITION

The child does not have to be able to stand, arms free, to attempt this item. (Review "standing" and "arms free" in the Explanation of Terms, pp 125–6, 128.) As mentioned in the Equipment section (p 44), the steps should be standard-sized. The therapist should be behind the child to minimize the possibility of injury. Position the child comfortably in standing at the base of the stairs holding on to one rail with one or two hands.

INSTRUCTIONS

This item may require several "test trials" to determine how many steps will be attempted and whether the child will be instructed to alternate legs.

The child must move one leg at a time and both legs must move up each step in order to receive credit for the required number of steps. Children who move one leg up one step and then bring the opposite leg up to the same step at any time during the four steps would only meet the criterion for a score of 2.

The child may hold on to the rail with one or two hands, but must take the majority of the weight through the legs.

*85. Standing, holding one rail: Walks down four steps, holding one rail, alternating feet

    0. does not initiate walking down steps, holding rail
    1. walks down 2 steps, holding rail, same foot leads consistently
    2. walks down 4 steps, holding rail, alternating feet inconsistently
    3. walks down 4 steps, holding rail, alternating feet

STARTING POSITION

Position the child comfortably in standing at the top of the stairs, holding on to one rail with one or two hands. The child does not have to be able to stand, arms free, to attempt this item. As mentioned in the Equipment section (p 44), the steps should be standard-sized. The therapist should be in front of the child to minimize the possibility of injury.

INSTRUCTIONS
This item may require several "practice" trials to determine how many steps will be attempted and whether the child will be instructed to alternate legs.

The child must move one leg at a time and both legs must move down each step in order to receive credit for the required number of steps. Children who move one leg down one step and then bring the opposite leg down to the same step at any time during the four steps would only meet the criterion for a score of 2.

The child may hold on to the rail with one or two hands, but must take the majority of the weight through the legs.

*86. <u>Standing: Walks up four steps, alternating feet</u>

     0. does not initiate walking up steps, arms free
     1. walks up 2 steps, same foot leads consistently
     2. walks up 4 steps, alternating feet inconsistently
     3. walks up 4 steps, alternating feet

STARTING POSITION
The child must be able to stand and walk, arms free, to attempt this item. Position the child comfortably in standing, arms free, at the base of the stairs. (Review "arms free" in the Explanation of Terms, p 128.) As mentioned in the Equipment section (p 44), the steps should be standard-sized. The therapist should be behind the child to minimize the possibility of injury.

INSTRUCTIONS
This item may require several "practice" trials to determine how many steps will be attempted and whether the child will be instructed to alternate legs.

The child must move one leg at a time and both legs must move up each step in order to receive credit for the required number of steps. Children who move one leg up one step and then bring the opposite leg up to the same step at any time during the four steps would only meet the criterion for a score of 2.

The child may not touch the rail or the steps with either hand (*i.e.* must remain arms free).

*87. <u>Standing: Walks down four steps, alternating feet</u>

    0. does not initiate walking down steps, arms free
    1. walks down 2 steps, same foot leads consistently
    2. walks down 4 steps, alternating feet inconsistently
    3. walks down 4 steps, alternating feet

STARTING POSITION
Position the child comfortably in standing, arms free at the top of the stairs. (Review "arms free" in the Explanation of Terms, p 128.) The child must be able to stand and walk, arms free, to attempt this item. As mentioned in the Equipment section (p 44), the steps should be standard-sized. The therapist should be in front of the child to minimize the possibility of injury.

INSTRUCTIONS
This item may require several "practice" trials to determine how many steps will be attempted and whether the child will be instructed to alternate legs.

The child must walk down the stairs one leg at a time and both legs must move down each step in order to receive credit for the required number of steps. Children who move one leg down one step and then bring the opposite leg down to the same step at any time during the four steps would only meet the criterion for a score of 2.

The child may not touch the rail or the steps with either hand (*i.e.* must remain arms free).

*88. <u>Standing on 15 cm (6 in) step: Jumps off, both feet simultaneously</u>

    0. does not initiate jumping off step, both feet simultaneously
    1. jumps off, both feet simultaneously, but falls
    2. jumps off, both feet simultaneously, but uses hands on floor to avoid falling
    3. jumps off, both feet simultaneously

STARTING POSITION
The child must be able to stand, arms free, to attempt this item. Position the

child comfortably in standing, arms free, on a step that is 15 cm (6 in) high. This may be on a stable bench 15 cm (6 in) high or the bottom step of the set of stairs (although the step may be closer to 18 cm (7 in) if it is standard-sized). (Review "standing" and "arms free" in the Explanation of Terms, pp 125–6, 128.)

INSTRUCTIONS
Instruct the child to jump off the step, both feet simultaneously. (Review "both feet simultaneously" in the Explanation of Terms, p 127.)

To obtain a score of 3, the child must jump off the step, both feet simultaneously, without falling and without using either arm on the floor to prevent falling.

To obtain a score of 2, the child must jump off the step, both feet simultaneously, but touching the floor with one or both hands is acceptable to avoid falling.

To obtain a score of 1, the child must jump off the step both feet simultaneously but cannot maintain enough balance on landing (even using arms on the floor) to avoid falling.

EXPLANATION OF TERMS

LYING

SUPINE
- lying on the back
- spine is in contact with the weight-bearing surface
- head and extremities may be in any position unless specified otherwise

PRONE
- lying on the abdomen
- abdomen and pelvis are in contact with the weight-bearing surface
- head and extremities may be in any position unless specified otherwise

SITTING

SITTING
- the ability to support the body "more or less upright" with weight on the buttocks. If the child is leaning far enough in any direction that propping with the arms is used, the elbow must be off the weight-bearing surface (*e.g.* bench, mat or floor). Otherwise the child would not be upright enough to be considered "sitting". As well leaning further back than 45° off upright in any direction would not be considered "sitting".
- includes any sitting position (including "W" sit) unless described otherwise (*e.g.* item 31 "with feet in front")

"W" SITTING
- weight is on both ischium and posterior medial aspect of both thighs
- hips are internally rotated with knees flexed in front so that each foot is lateral to the corresponding hip joint
- the lower leg may be rotated internally with weight on the anterior and lateral aspect of the lower leg and foot or rotated externally with weight on the anterior and medial aspect of the lower leg and foot

SIDE-SITTING (RIGHT)
- weight is well over the right ischium with both legs flexed to the left side and both feet close to or in line with the left hip

SITTING FEET SUPPORTED
- child is seated on a bench with hips and knees flexed at 90° and feet resting on the floor or a small bench

SITTING FEET FREE
- child is seated on a bench with hips and knees flexed at 90° and feet dangling without any support

4 POINT

4 POINT

- weight bearing on the hands and knees
- head, trunk and pelvis must be off the weight-bearing surface and/or the lower legs
- alignment, particularly of the arms and legs, may vary within the above limitations

CREEP

- to move in prone using the extremities, with the abdomen on the weight bearing surface
- includes any variation of commando crawling

CRAWL

- move on hands and knees
- arms and legs do not have to move alternately

HITCH

- to move jerkily
- may include "bunny hopping" or "bottom hitching" where the child moves forward using arms and/or legs while maintaining some variation of sitting

CRAWL RECIPROCALLY

- move on hands and knees with alternating movements of both the arms and the legs (these alternating movements do not necessarily need to be coordinated)
- "bunny hopping" and "bottom hitching" are not acceptable

KNEELING

HIGH KNEELING

- weight bearing on the knees
- alignment may vary as long as the buttocks are clear of the lower legs and/or the weight-bearing surface

HALF KNEELING

- weight bearing is on one knee and the opposite foot
- alignment may vary as long as the buttocks are clear of the lower legs and/or the weight-bearing surface

KNEEL WALK

- walk on the knees
- one step forward includes the movement of one leg from "push off" to floor contact

STANDING

STANDING

- being in the upright position on the feet
- alignment, particularly of the trunk and lower extremities, may vary

- alignment may also vary depending on whether or not the child is holding on and whether it is with one or both hands

SQUAT
- crouching close to the ground
- for purposes of this measure, both the hips/waist and knees must be flexed to >90°

KICK
- foot must be clear of the floor when the ball is contacted
- ball must move from impact of the foot

STAND ON ONE FOOT
- opposite foot must be clear of the floor

WALKING & RUNNING

CRUISE ONE STEP
- movement sideways of both legs (one at a time)

WALK FORWARD ONE STEP
- movement forward of one leg from push-off to floor contact or heel strike

WALK BACKWARD ONE STEP
- movement backward of one leg from push-off to floor contact

CONSECUTIVE STEPS
- without interruption
- pauses between steps must not be longer than 2 seconds
- see additional comments in items 73 and 74

RUN
- there must be an instant where both feet are off the floor at the same time (to distinguish running from walking quickly)

WALK QUICKLY
- both feet may be on the floor at the same time even though it is very brief

WALK UP ONE STEP
- child must move one leg at a time and both legs must have walked up one step

HOPPING & JUMPING

JUMP
- both feet must clear the floor

How to decide whether to use the GMFM-88 or the GMFM-66

The *GMFM-88* has 22 more items than the GMFM-66 and therefore provides more description of a child's motor abilities, especially in the development of early motor skills. It may be the measure of choice for children with severe motor disability, as is characteristic of children in GMFCS level V (see Appendix 1) and young children functioning primarily in the Lying & Rolling dimension. If the assessment of aids or orthoses is of interest it is necessary to use the GMFM-88. The GMFM-88 may be the measure to use if you are *not* interested in comparing change *between* children but are interested in describing abilities at one point in time or in measuring change in an individual child over time where the interval nature of the scale is not of concern. The GMFM-88 may be the choice if you do not have access to a computer to run the GMAE scoring program necessary to analyse the data from the GMFM-66.

The *GMFM-66* will be the measure of choice for research purposes, where the interval properties of the scale are of paramount importance. This would be the case, for example, when you want to judge, on a common scale, the change made by different children, or to follow a single child over time to compare the amount of change in common time frames. The GMFM-66 scoring also provides a measure of the standard error around each total score that greatly facilitates the interpretation of change.

There are also many clinical advantages to using the GMFM-66. The GMFM-66 has fewer items and has a method for obtaining a score for a child even in the event that not all items have been assessed. It will therefore require less time to administer and will allow you to target the child's current functional abilities. If children are cognitively impaired or have difficulty understanding what is expected of them, or if children refuse to try items (especially items that are far below their ability level), they will not be penalized in the GMFM-66 scoring as is the case with the GMFM-88 scoring. The GMFM-66 requires assessment data to be entered into a user-friendly computer program. The program provides displays of the data in several formats useful for both research and clinical purposes. These include a summary of the child's assessment information, a plot of GMFM-66 scores over multiple assessments, and the choice to display two versions of an item map (the picture of items displayed in order of difficulty or the picture of items displayed in the order they appear on the GMFM score sheet). The plot of a child's GMFM-66 score and the individual item responses on the item map should improve the interpretability of a child's score and allow therapists readily to see which items the child has accomplished, which items are close to the child's ability level and what are the emerging skills. This should be helpful for treatment planning.

Interpreting scores from the GMFM-88

Information on administering and scoring items for the GMFM-88 is found in Chapter 5. Individual item scores are recorded on the GMFM-88 score sheet and percent scores can be calculated for each of the five dimensions as well as a total score (which is the average of the five dimensions). A "Goal Total" score may also be calculated and can help to increase the responsiveness of the measure by narrowing the focus to include selected GMFM dimensions most relevant to the child's goals. For example, Susie is just under 2 years old and we can see from her first GMFM-88 assessment (Fig. A3.1, p 183) that she is initiating crawling. She has developed independent sitting skills and is just beginning to pull to stand on furniture. Based on her age, her interests and her skill level, her family and therapist would like her to work on her skills in these areas. Her goal areas on the GMFM-88 are therefore likely to be in the three dimensions of (1) Sitting, (2) Crawling & Kneeling, and (3) Standing.

The GMFM-88 was developed and validated using principles of classical test theory. Like most clinical measures in medicine, the data derived from the GMFM-88 are ordinal. Ordinal data are ordered but the distance between numbers is not equal even though the numbers imply that they are. For example, the scoring of individual items on the GMFM is 0, 1, 2 or 3. A person gets equal credit for moving from 0 to 1, 1 to 2 and 2 to 3. If one looks at the criterion for each of the scores, it can be seen that 0 is defined as not being able to initiate the task; 1 defines initiating but completing less than 10% of the task; 2 is defined as partially completing the task and spans anywhere from completing greater than 10% of the task to less than 100% task completion; and 3 is reserved for task completion. The order of increasing difficulty is built into the scoring but we know intuitively (and now empirically from the Rasch analysis) that the distances between 0 and 1, 1 and 2, and 2 and 3 are not equal either within or between items.

Summary scores for the GMFM-88 are derived by calculating the scores for each dimension of the GMFM and then averaging across dimensions. A total score in itself has limited meaning because although it represents a percentage of the items passed, there is no way to know which items have been accomplished unless one looks at the individual item scores.

Appendix 4 provides tables of GMFM-88 scores and GMFM-66 scores for a sample of 652 children with cerebral palsy by age group and GMFCS category (Tables A4.1 and A4.2, pp 205, 206). Change scores for these children over 6 month and 12 month periods are also provided to give an indication of the change and variability in change scores for a group of children who were followed as part of a longitudinal study of motor development (Tables A4.3 and A4.4, pp 207, 208). The children received a variety of interventions but primarily physical therapy.

While many people argue that ordinal measures give results similar to measures that have interval properties, this may not always be the case. In fact when trying to assess change over time as we do to evaluate treatment, data from ordinal measures may actually under- or overestimate change. (See Chapter 2 for a more thorough discussion of this issue.) Rasch analysis of the GMFM was done to overcome some of the limitations in scoring and interpretation of the GMFM-88.

Interpreting GMFM-66 scores—the Gross Motor Ability Estimator (GMAE) scoring program

In order to interpret scores for the GMFM-66 a computer program is required. This scoring program is called the Gross Motor Ability Estimator (GMAE), so named because it provides an estimate of the child's gross motor ability based on the child's scores on the GMFM items entered. This estimate, or GMFM-66 score, differs from the GMFM-88 score in that it has interval (as opposed to ordinal) properties.

132

Both the clinical and research options within the GMAE program allow the user to enter all of the original GMFM-88 items, or just the 66 items used to compute the GMFM-66 score. An advantage of the GMFM-66 is that it is possible to obtain an estimate of a child's score using only a subsample of the 66 items. Scoring the GMFM-88 requires that for any item not attempted the child receive a score of 0. In contrast the GMFM-66 allows the user to enter an item that is not attempted as "Not tested" or "Missing", and the program will calculate the child's ability based upon the scores actually tested and entered. *It is important to note, however, that the more GMFM-66 items that are completed, the more accurate the estimated score.* In a simulation analysis, it was demonstrated that an accurate estimate of a child's ability could be made with as few as 13 items; however, this has not been empirically tested, and guidelines are not available about the most appropriate subset of items to test. It would seem to make sense that if one were limited by time or in the number of items that could be administered, one should test as many items as possible around the child's current ability level (*e.g.* where there is variation in scores of 0, 1, 2 and 3), similar to obtaining basal and ceiling scores with other measures. For further discussion see the section "How many items do I need to test?" at the end of this chapter.

The GMAE program has a self-contained tutorial. A copy of the tutorial is found in Appendix 2. What follows here is an explanation of the way to use and interpret the output provided by the GMAE for the GMFM-66. The next section will be most useful after people have worked through the tutorial and become familiar with the computer program.

Interpreting the output from "Entering Individual Data from GMFM Score Sheets" into the GMAE program

GMFM-66 scores are obtained by entering the GMFM item scores into the program either individually for each child or as an ASCII (text only) batch file containing GMFM scores for multiple children. The option to enter the GMFM scores individually into the program was designed for clinical evaluation of children and to track their progress over time. In this program scores are retained in a database for future reference, and plots of progress are available within the program.

The second option, to input the scores into the GMAE program from an ASCII file, was designed with the researcher in mind. The program allows GMFM-66 scores to be calculated for large samples by saving data from a database/statistical package such as the Statistical Package for the Social Sciences (SPSS) into an ASCII or text file and reading it into the program. The research version provides a GMFM-66 score and the standard error of measurement of the score but does not allow the plotting of scores on an item map.

Once individual GMFM data are entered into the GMAE program, the client information is summarized in several ways.

ASSESSMENT INFORMATION SCREEN
The "assessment information screen" is the location where the GMFM-88 or GMFM-66 scores are entered. Once scores have been entered *and saved* there is an option to compute the GMFM-88 percent scores (but only when the 88-item option has been chosen and all 88 items entered). Otherwise the option is to compute the GMFM-66 score. In the top right

of the screen an estimate of the child's GMFM-66 score will be displayed along with the standard error of measurement (SEM) of the child's score and the 95% confidence intervals around the child's score (95% CI = ±1.96 × SEM). The SEM is unique for each GMFM-66 score. This method of calculating the SEM for each GMFM-66 score is more rigorous than with many tests that provide only one estimate of the standard error for all scores on the test; however, the SEM still does not account for all sources of error. The confidence intervals give an indication that a child's score is highly (95%) likely to fall somewhere between the lower and upper bound of this confidence interval. (For more information about SEMs, see Appendix 5.)

Referring to the GMFM-66 print-out for Susie (Figs A3.3, A3.4, pp 193, 194), the scores for her initial GMFM assessment give a GMFM-66 score of 41.61. The 95% confidence interval of 39.38–43.84 means that Susie's true score is highly likely to be somewhere between the lower bound of 39.38 and the upper bound of 43.84. This confidence interval is particularly useful when looking at change in a child's score over time to determine if the score has changed a significant amount more than would be expected by chance. Even though a child's score may change, when the confidence intervals around the two scores overlap, the change may be due to measurement variability or error as opposed to a true functional change (*e.g.* variability associated with the child's behaviour day to day). For example, upon reassessment six months later (Figs A3.5, A3.6, pp 195, 196), Susie has a GMFM-66 score of 44.97 with the 95% CI ranging from 42.89 to 47.05. Because the lower bound of the time 2 assessment (42.89) overlaps with the upper bound of the time 1 assessment (43.84) in this example we could *not* be sure that the change was more than that due to measurement variability. The program also displays the number of items that have been tested in order to calculate the GMFM-66 score.

ITEM MAPS

Item maps can be displayed from the Assessment Information Screen by clicking "Item Maps" from the top tool bar or from the Case Summary Screen at the bottom of the page. Both of these pages provide an option to view two item maps: (1) Item Map by Difficulty Order, and (2) Item Map by Item Order. Depending on the purpose it may be appropriate to look at one or both of the item maps.

What is an item map?

Item maps or "variable maps" provide a visual display of the difficulty estimates for items in a measure. These difficulty estimates can be visually displayed in a number of different formats. (For further elaboration of the different methods see Appendix 6.) Figure A7.1 (p 216) illustrates one format used for the GMFM-66, where the dimensions of the GMFM are listed along the vertical axis and the difficulty estimates are spread out along the horizontal axis by item number with the "steps" or response options (for GMFM these are 0, 1, 2 or 3) for all items indicated in different shading. The horizontal axis ranges from 0 to 100, where the items closer to 0 are easier and the items closer to 100 are more difficult. While this clearly shows the overall spread of items and response options, it is not possible to identify the specific item titles without looking them up on the score sheet or in the

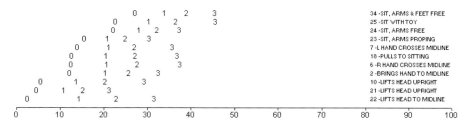

Fig. 6.1. Depiction of part of the "item map by difficulty order" for the GMFM-66.

manual. Another way to display item difficulties is shown in Figure A7.2 (p 217), in which the 50% and 90% probabilities of scoring a 3 for each GMFM-66 item are displayed.

An alternative method of displaying an item map (and the method that is used in the GMAE scoring program) is shown in Figures A3.3 and A3.5 (pp 193, 195). The item descriptions are arranged along the vertical axis and the available response options for each item are spread out horizontally beside that item according to difficulty level, with the easiest score (0) on the left and the hardest score (3) on the right. This map illustrates the location of the "expected scores" for each score (0, 1, 2, 3) for each item. We chose this method of displaying the item scores to be consistent with several other pediatric measures such as the Pediatric Evaluation of Disability Inventory (Haley *et al.* 1992) and the School Function Assessment (Coster *et al.* 1998). The expected score is "expected" in the sense that, if a large group of children of the same ability were tested, it indicates where their *mean* score on the item should be. For instance, looking at Figure 6.1, part of the item map by difficulty order, we can see that for item 22, 2 is the expected score for a GMFM-66 ability score of 23. This expected score indicates that if we tested a large number of children, all with a GMFM-66 score of 23, then their average score on the item should be a 2. (For an in-depth discussion of expected scores, refer to Appendix 6.)

Item maps can be useful to aid in the clinical interpretation of assessment scores for individual children assessed with the GMFM-66. The GMFM-66 item map is the best representation of GMFM item difficulty for children with cerebral palsy, regardless of type (*e.g.* spastic, dystonic, ataxic, hypotonic), limb distribution (*e.g.* hemiplegia, diplegia, quadriplegia) or GMFCS level. *Note that it is not appropriate to use this map for children with diagnoses other than cerebral palsy.*

Another approach to displaying the item response difficulties is presenting the items in the order that they are listed on the GMFM-66 score sheet, "Item Map by Item Order" (see Figs A3.4, A3.6, pp 194, 196). This format displays items in a way that is similar to the GMFM-88 "dimension" listing.

How do I interpret a GMFM-66 item map?
The difficulty of each GMFM-66 item is the same whether one is looking at the item map by *item order* or *difficulty order*. The same is true of the degree of difficulty to move between response options within an item. The only difference between these two maps is the order in which the items are displayed on the vertical axis.

135

• Figure A3.3 (p 193) shows the *item map by difficulty order* for Susie's initial GMFM assessment. The GMFM items are listed along the vertical (*y*) axis, and the horizontal (*x*) axis represents the total GMFM-66 scores. The most difficult item (#83: "Stands on left foot: Hops on left foot 10 times within a 60 cm (24 in) circle") is at the top left hand corner, and the easiest item (#22: "Sit on mat, supported at thorax by therapist: Lifts head to midline") is at the bottom right hand corner. Solely for display purposes, the items have been split so that the harder items are on the left and the easier items on the right, in order to format all this information on one page and allow the item names to be printed across from the appropriate item response options. The item numbers are the same as on the GMFM score sheet, but the item titles have been abbreviated to save space. If you are unsure of the full item title, refer to the GMFM manual or GMFM score sheet.

The difficulty of achieving a score of 0, 1, 2 or 3 within any GMFM item is displayed on the same line as the GMFM item number and name. If you take a ruler and draw a line across from any item, you can tell how difficult it is to move between the response options within that item by how far apart the numbers (0, 1, 2 and 3) are spaced. See, for example, item 79, "Stand: Kicks ball with left foot" (the 15th item from the top). The response options are fairly evenly spaced, indicating that the difficulty of moving from "initiates" (a score of 1) to "partially completes" (a score of 2), or from a score of 2 ("partially completes") to "completes" (a score of 3), is about the same. If we take another example (the item situated immediately below item 79 on the item map by difficulty order), item 57: "Stand: Lifts left foot, arms free 10 seconds", the distance between the response options is again fairly even indicating the difficulty in moving from a score of 1 to 2 or from 2 to 3 is again about the same. However, here the response options are much more spread out along the difficulty continuum, indicating that the degree of difficulty to go from a score of 1 ("initiating") ("lifts foot <3 seconds") to a score of 3 ("completing") on item 57 is much greater than moving from a 1 ("initiates kicking") to a 3 ("kicks the ball") on item 79. The difficulty of the items and the difficulty of the response options are both fixed and will not change whether you are looking at the item difficulty map or the item order map. The response options that are circled (in red on your monitor, and in red on the printout if you have a colour printer) indicate the actual scores that the child received on each item.

The horizontal (*x*) axis represents the GMFM-66 score on a scale ranging from 0 to 100. The information from Susie's initial GMFM-88 assessment was entered into the GMAE program and her item maps are presented in Figures A3.3 and A3.4 (pp 193, 194). Susie has a GMFM-66 score of 41.61. This has been plotted on the item map with the 95% confidence interval around the score indicated by the dotted lines. This score is the best estimate of this child's ability on the GMFM.

A few words should be added about the confidence intervals and expected scores. The confidence intervals indicate *how precisely* we can pinpoint a child's ability, not *how likely* a child is to achieve any specific item score. They are most useful for assessing whether or not a child has had a significant change in ability since a previous assessment, or to determine if the abilities of two children differ significantly.

The individual response option scores (0, 1, 2, 3) falling on the solid vertical line (at a score of just over 41) and within the 95% confidence intervals indicate what Susie may be expected to score based on her total GMFM-66 score. Scores to the left of the line are items Susie is likely to have accomplished, and scores to the right of the line are those that may be expected in the future. The responses circled in red are Susie's actual scores. By displaying the *item map by difficulty order* (Fig. A3.3, p 193) you are able to see clearly where Susie is functioning and what the next emerging skills are likely to be. The scores closer to the line on the right-hand side should be relatively easier for Susie than those item scores further away from the line on the right side.

Susie has some variability of scores both to the left and to the right of the line indicated as her total GMFM-66 score of 41.61; however, she does not have any scores that are really unexpected. If Susie had scored less than a 3 on items 21 (sit: lifts head upright) and 22 (sit: lifts head to midline) then it would be important to look at these items in more detail as these are the easiest items on the GMFM-66. Based on Susie's total GMFM-66 score it would be predicted that Susie would easily be able to accomplish these items. Scores for items 21 and 22 are not circled on this item map because these items were not actually tested (and therefore were entered as "missing" into the GMAE program). If in fact Susie truly did score 0 on these two items, it would be important to look at this more closely as it may indicate an issue with head control. Looking up the difficulty scale you can see that Susie starts scoring zeros more consistently at item 65, and continues to score zeros on the remaining more difficult items (with the exception of scores of 1 for items 45 and 35). What is not immediately clear from the item difficulty map is how Susie has performed in the different dimensions of the GMFM. To look at this question in more detail, we may wish to look at the *item map by item order* (Fig. A3.4, p 194) to see if there is any pattern to the items.

• Figure A3.4 (p 194) shows the *item map by item order* for Susie's initial assessment. This lists the GMFM items on the vertical (y) axis in the order they appear on the GMFM score sheet, starting with items in Lying & Rolling in the top right-hand corner and ending with items in the Walking, Running & Jumping dimension in the lower left corner. The difficulty and spacing of the response options within items have not changed from the item map by difficulty order (Fig. A3.3, p 193). The horizontal (x) axis displays the possible GMFM-66 scores, ranging from 0 to 100. Again, the child's score is represented as a solid vertical line, with the dotted lines indicating the 95% confidence intervals around the score.

It can be seen that Susie is capable of all items in Lying & Rolling, has variability in scores through the Sitting and Crawling & Kneeling dimensions, is just beginning to initiate pulling to stand, and is unable to initiate any of the Walking, Running & Jumping activities.

If you choose to display the item map by item order, it may be easier to see what a child is accomplishing within different dimensions (*e.g.* "Sitting") as those items will be listed together. The emerging skills across dimensions may be harder to discern from this map because the difficulty of items is no longer ordered.

CASE SUMMARY SCREEN
In addition to the client information (name, gender, birth date, diagnosis) the Case Summary Screen shows a plot of the child's GMFM-66 score. If multiple assessments for the same

client are entered, all the assessments can be plotted on the same graph (Fig. A3.7, p 197). The following information for multiple assessments will also be available in an integrated table: the assessment dates; age at each assessment; GMFM-66 scores; SEM; lower and upper boundary of the 95% confidence interval; number of items tested; GMFCS level; the name of the assessing therapist; and the change score from the previous assessment.

Contrasting the various scoring methods

As you may recall, at Susie's initial GMFM-88 assessment both her parents and her therapist were pleased with her progress but were uncertain about what the total scores meant and what they could expect Susie to accomplish over the next several months. Let's look at the different ways Susie's score may be expressed. From the information provided in Figures A3.1 and A3.2 (pp 185, 191):

GMFM-88 Time 1 score = 32%

GMFM-88 Time 2 score = 43%

Change in GMFM-88 = 11%

In reviewing the data from the original 88-item GMFM assessments that were done with Susie, we need to scan the original GMFM score sheet to see both what she could and could not do on each occasion, and what items showed progress over the six months from April to October 1989. We note that she had made most of her progress in the Crawling & Kneeling dimension, where she was showing progress in the 4-point skills (items 41, 43–46) that are thought to be important for prone mobility. Her score within that dimension changed from 15 to 25. Her score also increased in the Sitting dimension, from 33 to 39. Item review showed that she was more secure in sitting (*e.g.* items 21, 22 and 32) and she showed improvement in items relating to sitting on a bench or chair (28, 29, and 35–37). (However, it should be noted that Susie had refused to attempt several items at both initial and repeat assessments that would have negatively impacted on her score.) It is also noteworthy that there is no way to compare the magnitude of change (10 points) in Crawling & Kneeling with the magnitude of change (6 points) in Sitting.

Figure A3.8 (pp 198–203) is an example of how the new GMFM score sheet would be completed using Susie's repeat assessment. The items Susie refused to attempt are now indicated as "Not Tested" (NT). Susie's GMFM-88 score would not change; however, this information would be used in the GMAE program for the calculation of her GMFM-66 score.

We could also try to understand Susie's score in relation to what other children with cerebral palsy of a similar age and a similar level of motor ability might score. Again, when Susie was first seen her "severity" of motor disability was assessed using the clinical judgment of her physical therapist. Today, she could be assessed with the GMFCS. If we judge that Susie has a GMFCS level III, we could look at Table A4.3 (p 207) and see that for a child of 2–4 years of age we might expect a change in her GMFM-88 score over 6 months of approximately 5%. Susie's change of 11% seems very positive in light of what might be expected for her age and GMFCS level.

Another way the information from the GMFM-88 could have been displayed to Susie's parents is by narrowing in on the areas identified by the family as being important. These goal areas are used to calculate a goal total score. For Susie's family these were Sitting,

Standing, and Walking, Running & Jumping. The goal total score showed a large change for Susie (16%) relative to her total GMFM-88 change score (11%):

GMFM Goal Total Time 1 = 31%
GMFM Goal Total Time 2 = 47%
Change in Goal Total = 16%

What is not clear with the GMFM-88, however, is the "meaning" of this amount of numerical change. Nor are we able to recognize from these findings what emerging aspects of function were more and less difficult, and what we might expect in the next several months. It is here that the GMFM-66 analyses are particularly helpful. Recognizing that the units of change in the total GMFM-66 score are "interval" rather than simply percentage changes enables us to see the changes differently.

Now we can observe from the item difficulty maps (Figs A3.3, A3.5, pp 193, 195) a change from a GMFM-66 score of 41.61 (95% CI = 39–44) to a score of 44 .97 (95% CI = 43–47) and can see that there is a slight overlap in the 95% confidence intervals. The amount of change on the GMFM-66 is numerically smaller (3.36 GMAE units) than that on the GMFM-88 (11%). More important, however, is that because of the overlapping confidence intervals we cannot be sure that the change is more than might be attributable to measurement error.

The second value of the item maps is to illustrate the relative distances between "steps" or response options within items, as these are spread out on the item map by difficulty order. Thus, for example, the "distance" from a score of 1 to a score of 3 on item 67 ("Stand, two hands held: walks forward 10 steps") is relatively small, whereas for item 80 ("Stand: Jumps 30 cm (12 in) high, both feet simultaneously") this distance is much greater. This information will be helpful in planning therapy and in tempering our expectations for change on each of these items. The item map by item order helps us to recognize what skills are likely to be emerging and to plan therapy and play activities in an effort to encourage the development of these "next" aspects of function.

Let us look at another example using Susie's GMFM-66 information (Figs A3.3–A3.6). Susie could not maintain a standing position even with both hands holding onto furniture (she scored a 0 on item 53) at her initial assessment. At reassessment she was able to maintain standing for at least 3 seconds while holding on with one hand (scoring a 2 on item 53). The response options for this item (#53) are spread out rather widely, indicating that a child needs a relatively large change in overall gross motor ability to move between a score of 0 and a score of 2. On the other hand, at her initial assessment Susie was beginning to crawl but could not go further than 60 cm (2 ft) for a score a 1 on item 44, whereas by the time of her reassessment she was able to crawl for 1.8 m (6 ft). We can tell by the spacing on the item map for item 44 that it is generally easier for children to crawl 1.8 m once they have commenced crawling than it is to move from standing with two hands holding furniture to standing independently. While the GMFM-88 score would give equal weight to the two-point change on both these items, it is clear from the item map that it is more difficult to complete item 53 than to complete item 44.

We know that Susie's change on the GMFM-66 over the six-month period between assessments was 3.36. As with the GMFM-88 score, it is possible to look at Tables A4.3

and A4.4 (pp 207, 208) to see what kind of change might be expected based on scores from other children of Susie's age with similar levels of gross motor abilities over 6 and 12 month intervals. Table A4.3 shows that children who are between 2 and 4 years of age and are at GMFCS level III had an average change score over 6 months of 2.43 on the GMFM-66. Susie's score is slightly above the mean score.

For more clinical examples of interpreting item maps, see Appendices 8 and 9.

Interpreting the output from the research version of the GMAE program
After entering a data file into the GMAE program for analysis, the output will include the child's name (or ID), the GMFM-66 score and the standard error of measurement around that score. It is not possible to get item maps or case summaries from data entered in this way. (For an example, see the "Research Section" of the GMAE tutorial in Appendix 2.)

Are scores from the GMFM-66 and GMFM-88 related?
It is not appropriate to compare GMFM-88 and GMFM-66 scores. The GMFM-88 is scored as a percentage of the total items completed, while the GMFM-66 is scored on a logit scale that has been transformed to scale from 0 to 100 but still retains the log-linear properties of a logit scale. Thus, even though the endpoints of both scales are the same the units are very different—this is clearly shown in Figure 2.1 (p 7).

In our example of Susie, the GMFM-88 score looks to be more responsive to change than the GMFM-66 score. Her change score using the GMFM-88 is 11%, but using the GMFM-66 score her change in score is only 3.36 GMAE units.

Now that we know that the GMFM-88 and GMFM-66 scores (and therefore change scores) may be numerically very different between the GMFM-88 and the GMFM-66, it is important to look at why that difference arises and what it means for the interpretation of the GMFM-66. We will continue to use the example of Susie.

At her first assessment Susie scored 41.61 on the GMFM-66 with a GMFM-88 percent score of 31%. Six months later Susie had improved and scored 45 on the GMFM-66 and 43% on the GMFM-88. The jump of 12% in the GMFM-88 score reflects the increase from a raw score of 82 to a raw score of 107—a net increase of 25 item scores. By examining the scoring differences between the GMFM-88 and the GMFM-66 we can get a better idea of why the change score for the two measures is so different for Susie over six months. To do this we will look at three components of the change score: (i) the change in item scores on the 22 items that have been removed and are no longer scored for the GMFM-66; (ii) the change in item scores on the GMFM-66 items; and (iii) the change in scores resulting from items not tested at one assessment. The net change in item scores on the 22 removed items was 7, resulting from an increase of 11 points and a decrease of four points on those items. This change was measured on items that are "noisy" (*i.e.* that do not reliably contribute to the underlying trait of gross motor function) and this change is not considered in computing the GMFM-66 score. This change is responsible for 3.5% of the change exhibited on the GMFM-88.

The second component of change not considered in the GMFM-66 is the part due to items that are refused during testing. The net change score resulting from the refusal of items was 1: five points were gained from refusing items at Time 1, and four points were lost for refusing items at Time 2. Because Susie was not penalized at either assessment for refusing items this change was not reflected in her GMFM-66 score.

That leaves the change due to the items that are scored in the GMFM-66. If we consider just these 66 items there is still a 17 point (8.5%) change score as measured by the GMFM-88 but only a 3.4 point change score as measured by the GMFM-66. The explanation for this difference can be seen in the schematic of the item step difficulties shown as Figure A7.1 (p 216). Susie's improvements are a result of the acquisition of new skills of similar difficulty or small improvements in existing skills. This type of improvement generally occurs when the child is functioning in the middle range of the scale (as Susie is with a GMFM-66 score of 41.61), where many skills are emerging simultaneously, as seen on the map where the items are clumped together. Improvements in function on a number of items of similar difficulty may "inflate" the GMFM-88 score because the child is doing, and receiving credit for, more activities; however, since these are emerging at roughly the same time in the child's development the GMFM-66 score will change relatively less that the GMFM-88 score. In this instance, Susie is fully able to attain the 4 point position and can reach and crawl from this position; by improving her ability to maintain the 4 point position she improves the scores of four items (41, 43, 44 and 46). With these items Susie is gaining important movements but instead of increasing the *difficulty level* of her movements she is *adding different movements of similar difficulty* to her functional repertoire. While the GMFM-88 gives credit for each new *movement*, the GMFM-66 attempts instead to credit each new *skill*.

A useful analogy of the difference between new movements and an increase in ability can be seen with a child learning to spell. Initially a child will learn the alphabet and then move on to simple words. The hurdle from the alphabet to a word is a significant one and should be credited. However, once the child has mastered simple words like "cat" and "dog", other similar words like "bat" and "hat" or "log" and "hog" should come easily, although it would require a new skill to master words where, for example, the presence of one vowel modified the sound of another, as in "cake" or "date" and yet another skill to master silent letters such as in "lamb". Imagine that the GMFM measured spelling ability with the above words. Using this analogy the GMFM-88 would give equal credit for "cat", "date" and "lamb". In contrast, the GMFM-66 would give some credit for "cat", more credit for "date" and even more credit for "lamb", but would not give very much extra credit if the child also got "hat" and "cake".

The difference in apparent responsiveness between the two measures can be highlighted using two children of different abilities. At the first assessment Sally can only spell "cat", while Toby can spell all the simple words plus "date" and "cake". Six weeks later Sally can spell "cat", "dog", "bat" and "hat" and Toby can now spell "lamb" (in addition to all the words he could spell previously). If the GMFM-88 were used to assess the change score, Sally's change would look much bigger because she would change three points, from a 1 to a 4, whereas Toby's score would improve only one point, from a 6 to a 7. If on the other hand the GMFM-66 were used then Sally's score would improve only marginally because her new words are of similar difficulty—on the item schematic in Appendix 7 (Fig. A7.1, p 216) these items would be closely stacked. Toby's scores would show a larger change on the GMFM-66 because his new word is of much greater difficulty than he had previously achieved.

How many items do I need to test?

There are no hard and fast rules about how many items are sufficient when administering the GMFM-66. However, using a computer simulation exercise we were able to determine the *absolute minimum* number of items required to determine the GMFM-66 score.

Ability levels for 100 subjects were simulated. These simulated ability levels were then used as the "true" ability levels for the subjects and according to methods proposed by Smith (1982) were used to simulate item responses which "fit" the Rasch model for children with cerebral palsy. A random selection of a specified number of items was then drawn and just these items were used to estimate the GMFM-66 score for each of 100 subjects. This estimated ability was then compared to the "true" ability using an intraclass correlation coefficient, ICC(1,1). This process was repeated for 100 simulations for each possible number of items tested (*i.e.* 1 to 66). The mean agreement between "true" and "estimated" abilities was then examined as a function of the number of items tested.

We found that the absolute minimum number of items required to estimate the true ability of a child 95 times out of 100 times is 13. It is tempting to want to assess the minimum number of items. However, we also know that the agreement between the true score and estimated score increases with the number of items tested. Furthermore, this was a simulation exercise and has not been empirically validated. Therefore, it is recommended that when possible, all items should be tested.

If I am limited in the number of items I have time to administer, how do I know which ones to choose?

It is important to test items around the child's current ability level. For example, if a child is scoring all 0's or all 3's on the items being tested then there is not enough information about the child's abilities and limitations to give a good estimate of their ability. The items tested should include items on which the child has some success (scores of 1 to 3) and some items that the child cannot complete (scores of 0). When the items cover the child's functional range the child can be more accurately located on the continuum of gross motor function.

of motor development at the extremes of childhood—of infants and toddler-aged children with CP, and of adolescents and young adults. In particular how do the patterns of very early development relate to later outcomes, with respect to both "activity" and "participation" (WHO 2001)? The predictive validity of the GMFCS for children below the age of 2 years remains somewhat limited (Palisano *et al.* 1997). This may be because there is relatively less information available in the somewhat restricted motor repertoire of the infant. Perhaps the early manifestations of the motor impairments that become CP are less stable than the patterns of older preschool and school-aged children. What is clear, not surprisingly, is that our ability to prognosticate about long-term motor outcomes improves as the child gets older (Wood and Rosenbaum 2000). To respond most effectively to the prime questions of parents of infants with CP, about the prognosis for their child's gross motor function, will require more work to study and chart carefully the motor development of infants.

REFERENCES

Abel M, Damiano D, Pannunzio M, Bush J (1997) 'Role of multiple muscle-tendon recessions and releases to improve motor function in diplegic cerebral palsy.' *Developmental Medicine and Child Neurology*, **39**, Suppl. 75, 16–17.

Almeida GL, Campbell SK, Girolami G, Penn R, Corcos DM (1997) 'Multidimensional assessment of motor function in a child with cerebral palsy following intrathecal administration of baclofen.' *Physical Therapy*, **77**, 751–764.

Avery LM, Russell DJ, Raina PS, Walter SD, Rosenbaum PL (2002) 'Rasch analysis of the Gross Motor Function Measure: Validating the assumptions of the Rasch model to create an interval level measure.' *Archives of Physical Medicine and Rehabilitation* (in press).

Bartlett DJ, Palisano RJ (2000) 'A multivariate model of determinants of motor change for children with cerebral palsy.' *Physical Therapy*, **80**, 598–614.

Barwood S, Baillieu C, Boyd R, Brereton K, Low J, Nattrass G, Graham HK (2000) 'Analgesic effects of botulinum toxin A: a randomized, placebo-controlled clinical trial.' *Developmental Medicine and Child Neurology*, **42**, 116–121.

Bayley N (1993) *Manual for the Bayley Scales of Infant Development, 2nd edn*. San Antonio, TX: Psychological Corporation.

Beckung E, Hagberg G (2002) 'Neuroimpairments, activity limitations and participation restrictions in children with cerebral palsy.' *Developmental Medicine and Child Neurology*, **44**, 309–316.

Bjornson KF, Graubert CS, McLaughlin JF, Astley SJ (1994) 'Inter-rater reliability of the Gross Motor Function Measure.' *Developmental Medicine and Child Neurology*, **36**, (Suppl 70), 27–28.

Bjornson KF, Graubert CS, Burford VL, McLaughlin JF (1998a) 'Validity of the Gross Motor Function Measure.' *Pediatric Physical Therapy*, **10** (2), 43–47.

Bjornson KF, Graubert CS, McLaughlin JF, Kerfeld CI, Clark EM (1998b) 'Test–retest reliability of the Gross Motor Function Measure in children with cerebral palsy.' *Physical and Occupational Therapy in Pediatrics*, **18** (2), 51–61.

Bleck EE (1975) 'Locomotor prognosis in cerebral palsy.' *Developmental Medicine and Child Neurology*, **17**, 18–25.

Bower E, McLellan D (1992) 'Effect of increased exposure to physiotherapy on skill acquisition of children with cerebral palsy.' *Developmental Medicine and Child Neurology*, **34**, 25–39.

Bower E, McLellan DL, Arney J, Campbell MJ (1996) 'A randomized controlled trial of different intensities of physiotherapy and different goal-setting procedures in 44 children with cerebral palsy.' *Developmental Medicine and Child Neurology*, **38**, 226–237.

Bower E, Michell D, Campbell M, McLellan D (2001) 'Randomized controlled trail of physiotherapy in 56 children with cerebral palsy followed for 18 months.' *Developmental Medicine and Child Neurology*, **43**, 4–15.

Boyce W, Gowland C, Rosenbaum P, Lane M, Plews N, Goldsmith C, Russell D, Wright V, Zdrobov S, Harding D (1995) 'The Gross Motor Performance Measure: validity and responsiveness of a measure of quality of movement.' *Physical Therapy*, **75**, 603–613.

Bryk AS, Raudenbush SW (1992) *Hierarchical Linear Models*. Newbury Park, CA: Sage.

Buckon CE, Sienko Thomas S, Jakobson-Huston S, Moor M, Sussman M, Aiona M (2001) 'Comparison of three ankle–foot orthosis configurations for children with spastic hemiplegia.' *Developmental Medicine and Child Neurology*, **43**, 371–378.

Campbell SK, Osten ET, Kolobe TA, Fisher AG (1993) 'Development of the Test of Infant Motor Performance.' *In:* Granger CV, Gresham GE (eds) *New Developments in Functional Assessment. Physical Medicine and Rehabilitation Clinics of North America*. Philadelphia: WB Saunders, pp 541–550.

Campbell Torpey P, Herrle, S (2000) 'Use of the S.W.A.S.H. orthosis for sitting and gait function in a child with sequelae of septic hip.' *Physical Therapy Case Reports*, **3** (2), 45–56.

Chambers LW, Haines T (1982) *Guide To Fundamentals Of Measurement In Health And Health Care Research/Evaluation*. Hamilton: McMaster University.

Coster W, Beeney T, Haltiwinger J, Haley SM (1998) *School Function Assessment*. San Antonio, TX:

Psychological Corporation/Therapy Skill Builders.

Cronk C, Crocker AC, Pueschel SM, Shea AM, Zackai E, Pickens G, Reed RB (1988) 'Growth charts for children with Down syndrome: 1 month to 18 years of age.' *Pediatrics*, **81**, 102–110.

Damiano DL, Abel MF (1996) 'Relation of gait analysis to gross motor function in cerebral palsy.' *Developmental Medicine and Child Neurology*, **38**, 389–396.

Damiano DL, Abel MF (1998) 'Functional outcomes of strength training in spastic cerebral palsy.' *Archives of Physical Medicine and Rehabilitation*, **79**, 119–125.

Damiano D, Martellotta T, Sullivan D, Granata K, Abel M (2000) 'Muscle force production and functional performance in spastic cerebral palsy: Relationship of cocontraction.' *Archives of Physical Medicine and Rehabilitation*, **81**, 895–900.

Deyo RA, Centor RM (1986) 'Assessing the responsiveness of functional scales to clinical change: An analogy to diagnostic test performance.' *Journal of Chronic Disease*, **39**, 897–906.

Deyo RA, Inui TS (1984) 'Toward clinical applications of health status measures: sensitivity of scales to clinically important changes.' *Health Services Research*, **19**, 275–289.

Drouin L, Malouin F, Richards C, Marcoux S (1996) 'Correlation between the Gross Motor Function Measure scores and gait spatiotemporal measures in children with neurological impairments.' *Developmental Medicine and Child Neurology*, **38**, 1007–1019

Evans C, Gowland C, Rosenbaum P, Willan A, Russell D, Weber D, Plews N (1994) 'The effectiveness of orthoses for children with cerebral palsy.' *Developmental Medicine and Child Neurology*, **36**, Suppl. 70, 26 (abstract).

Flett P, Stern L, Waddy H, Connell T, Seeger J, Gibson S (1999) 'Botulinum toxin A versus fixed cast stretching for dynamic calf tightness in cerebral palsy.' *Journal of Paediatrics and Child Health*, **35**, 71–77.

Folio R, Fewell R, DuBoise RF (1983) *Peabody Developmental Motor Scales and Activity Cards*. Allen, TX: DLM Teaching Resources.

Gemus M, Palisano R, Russell D, Rosenbaum P, Walter SD, Galuppi B, Lane M (2001) 'Using the Gross Motor Function Measure to evaluate motor development in children with Down syndrome.' *Physical and Occupational Therapy in Pediatrics*, **21**, 69–79.

Gill S, Curran A, Tripp J, Melarickas L, Hurran C, Stanley O (2001) 'Hyperkinetic movement disorder in an 11-year-old child treated with bilateral pallidal stimulators.' *Developmental Medicine and Child Neurology*, **43**, 350–353.

Guyatt G, Walter S, Norman G (1987) 'Measuring change over time: Assessing the usefulness of evaluative instruments.' *Journal of Chronic Disease*, **40**, 171–180.

Guyatt GH, Kirshner B, Jaeschke R (1992) 'Measuring health status: what are the necessary measurement properties?' *Journal of Clinical Epidemiology*, **12**, 1341–1345.

Haley SM, Coster WJ, Ludlow LH, Haltiwanger JT, Andrellos PJ (1992) *Pediatric Evaluation of Disability Inventory (PEDI). Development, Standardization and Administration Manual*. Boston: PEDI Research Group, New England Medical Center Hospitals.

Haley SM, McHorney CA, Ware JE (1994) 'Evaluation of the MOS SF-36 Physical Functioning Scale: I. Unidimensionality and reproducibilty of the Rasch scale.' *Journal of Clinical Epidemiology*, **47**, 671–684.

Handlesman D (1994) 'The construct validity of the Worker Role Interview for the Chronic Mentally Ill.' Masters thesis, University of Illinois at Chicago.

Harris T, Damiano D, Abel M (1997) 'Gait efficiency in diplegic cerebral palsy.' *Developmental Medicine and Child Neurology*, **39**, Suppl. 75, 28–29.

Hays R, Bjornson K, McLaughlin J, Astley K (1995) 'Selective dorsal rhizotomy: relationship of rootlet responses to clinical measures of spasticity and motor function.' *Developmental Medicine and Child Neurology*, **37**, Suppl. 73, 4 (abstract).

Hays R, McLaughlin J, Bjornson K, Stephens K, Roberts T, Price R (1998) 'Electrophysiological monitoring during selective dorsal rhizotomy, and spasticity and GMFM performance.' *Developmental Medicine and Child Neurology*, **40**, 233–238.

Hays R, Morales L, Reise S (2000) 'Item response theory and health outcomes measurement in the 21st century.' *Medical Care*, **38**, Suppl. 2, pII–28:II–42.

Hoskins TA, Squires JE (1973) 'Developmental assessment: A test for gross motor and reflex development.' *Physical Therapy*, **53**, 117–125.

Kaplan RM, Bush JW, Berry CC (1976) 'Health status: Types of validity and the index of well being.' *Health Services Research*, **11**, 478–506.

Kennes J, Rosenbaum P, Hanna SE, Walter S, Russell D, Raina P, Bartlett D, Galuppi B (2002) 'Health status of school-aged children with cerebral palsy: information from a population-based sample.' *Developmental Medicine and Child Neurology*, **44**, 240–247.

Kirshner B, Guyatt G (1985) 'A methodological framework for assessing health indices.' *Journal of Chronic Disease*, **38**, 27–36.

Kolobe TH, Palisano RJ, Stratford PW (1998) 'Comparison of two outcome measures for infants with cerebral palsy and infants with motor delay.' *Physical Therapy*, **78**, 1062–1072.

Krach L, Gilmartin R, Bruce D, Storrs B, Abbott R, Ward J, Bloom K, Brooks W, Madsen J, McLaughlin J, Nadell J (1997) 'Functional changes noted following treatment of individuals with cerebral palsy with intrathecal baclofen.' *Developmental Medicine and Child Neurology*, **39**, Suppl. 75, 12–13.

Kraemer HC, Karner AF (1976) 'Statistical alternatives in assessing quantitative measures: application to behavior measures of neonates.' *Psychological Bulletin,* **85**, 914–921.

Landgraf JM, Abetz L, Ware JE (1996) *Child Health Questionnaire (CHQ). A User's Manual.* Boston: The Health Institute, New England Medical Centre.

Lane M, Russell D (2002) *Gross Motor Function Measure (GMFM) self-instructional training program* [CD-ROM]. London: Mac Keith Press.

Law M, King G, MacKinnon E, Russell D, Murphy C, Hurley P (1999) *All About Outcomes: A program to help you understand, evaluate and choose pediatric outcome measures.* [CD-ROM]. Thorofare, NJ: Slack.

Li M, Olejnik S (1997) 'The power of Rasch person-fit statistics in detecting unusual response patterns.' *Applied Psychological Measurement*, **21**, 215–231.

Lim HH, Marriott DA, Potter PD, Clayton-Krasinski D (2000) 'Comparison of two methods of training student physical therapists to score the Gross Motor Function Measure.' *Pediatric Physical Therapy*, **12**, 127–132.

Linacre JM, Wright BD (1996) *A User's Guide to Bigsteps Rasch-Model Computer Program.* Chicago: MESA Press.

Lipsey MW (1983) 'A scheme for assessing measurement sensitivity in program evaluation and other applied research.' *Psychological Bulletin*, **94**, 152–265.

MacKinnon J, Noh S, Lariviere J, MacPhail A, Allan D, Laliberte D (1995) 'A study of therapeutic effects of horseback riding for children with cerebral palsy.' *Physical and Occupational Therapy in Pediatrics*, **15** (1), 17–31.

MacPhail A, Kramer J (1995) 'Effect of isokinetic strength training on functional ability and walking efficiency in adolescents with cerebral palsy.' *Developmental Medicine and Child Neurology*, **37**, 763–775.

Magalhaes L, Fisher A, Bernspang B, Linacre J (1996) 'Cross-cultural assessment of functional ability.' *Occupational Therapy Journal of Research*, **1**, 45–63.

Mahoney G, Robinson C, Fewell RR (2001) 'The effects of early motor intervention on children with Down syndrome or cerebral palsy: A field study.' *Journal of Developmental and Behavioral Pediatrics*, **22**, 153–162.

Mall V, Heinen F, Kirschner J, Linder M, Stein S, Michaelis U, Bernius P, Lane M, Korinthenberg R (2000) 'Evaluation of botulinum toxin A therapy in children with adductor spasm by Gross Motor Function Measure.' *Journal of Child Neurology*, **15**, 214–217.

Maltais D, Bar-Or O, Galea V, Pierrynowski M (2001) 'Use of orthoses lowers the O_2 cost of walking in children with spastic cerebral palsy.' *Medicine and Science in Sports and Exercise*, **33**, 320–325.

McBride MC, Laroia N, Guillet R (2000) 'Electrographic seizures in neonates correlate with poor neuro-developmental outcome.' *Neurology*, **55**, 506–513.

McDowell I, Newell C (1987) *Measuring Health.* Oxford: Oxford University Press.

McLaughlin J, Bjornson K, Graubert C, Pong A, Hays R, Hoffinger S (1991) 'Ability to detect functional change with the Gross Motor Function Measure: a pilot study.' *Developmental Medicine and Child Neurology*, **33**, Suppl. 64, 26 (abstract).

McLaughlin J, Bjornson K, Astley S, Hays R, Hoffinger S, Aramantrout E, Roberts T (1994) 'The role of selective dorsal rhizotomy in cerebral palsy: critical evaluation of a prospective clinical series.' *Developmental Medicine and Child Neurology*, **36**, 755–769.

McLaughlin J, Bjornson K, Astley S, Hays R, Roberts TS, Graubert C, Temkin N, Dales M, Hoffinger S (1996) 'Efficacy of selective dorsal rhizotomy in cerebral palsy: changes in mobility after 12 months.' *Developmental Medicine and Child Neurology*, **38**, Suppl. 74, 4 (abstract).

McLaughlin J, Bjornson K, Astley S, Hays R, Price R, Roberts TS, Graubert C, Temkin N, Song K, Dales M (1997) 'Efficacy of selective dorsal rhizotomy in spastic diplegia: changes in mobility after 24 months.' *Developmental Medicine and Child Neurology*, **39**, Suppl. 75, 15 (abstract).

McLaughlin J, Bjornson K, Astley S, Graubert C, Hays R, Roberts T, Price R, Temkin N (1998) 'Selective dorsal rhizotomy: efficacy and safety in an investigator-masked randomized clinical trial.' *Developmental*

Medicine and Child Neurology, **40**, 220–232.

Meenan RF, Anderson JJ, Kazis LE, Egger MJ, Altz-Smith M, Samuelson CO, Willkens RF, Solsky MA, Hayes SP, Blocka KL, Weinstein A, Guttadauria M, Kaplan SB, Klippel J (1984) 'Outcome assessment in clinical trials: Evidence for the sensitivity of a health status measure.' *Arthritis and Rheumatism*, **27**, 1344–1352.

Mitchell SK (1979) 'Interobserver agreement, reliability, and generalizability of data collected in observational studies.' *Psychological Bulletin*, **86**, 376–390.

Molenaar I, Hoijtinik H (1990) 'The many null distribution of person fit indices.' *Psychometrika*, **55**, 75–106.

Mulligan H, Climo K, Hanson C, Mauga P (1999) 'Physiotherapy treatment intensity for a child with cerebral palsy: a single case study.' *New Zealand Journal of Physiotherapy*, **28** (2), 6–12.

Mutch L, Alberman E, Hagberg B, Kodama K, Velickovic M (1992) 'Cerebral palsy epidemiology: where are we now and where are we going?' *Developmental Medicine and Child Neurology*, **34**, 547–555.

Nordmark E, Jarnlo GB, Hagglund G (2000) 'Comparison of the Gross Motor Function Measure and Paediatric Evaluation of Disability Inventory in assessing motor function in children undergoing selective dorsal rhizotomy.' *Developmental Medicine and Child Neurology*, **42**, 245–252.

Nordmark E, Hagglund G, Jarnlo GB (1997) 'Reliability of the Gross Motor Function Measure in cerebral palsy.' *Scandinavian Journal of Rehabilitative Medicine*, **29**, 25–28.

Norusis MJ (1986) *SPSSX version 2.1*. Chicago: SPSS.

Nunnally JC (1978) *PsychometricTheory, 2nd edn*. New York: McGraw-Hill.

Palisano R, Rosenbaum P, Walter S, Russell D, Wood E, Galuppi B (1997) 'Development and validation of a gross motor function classification system for children with cerebral palsy.' *Developmental Medicine and Child Neurology*, **39**, 214–223.

Palisano RJ, Hanna SE, Rosenbaum PL, Russell DJ, Walter SD, Wood EP, Raina PS, Galuppi BE (2000) 'Validation of a model of gross motor function for children with cerebral palsy.' *Physical Therapy*, **80**, 974–985.

Palisano RJ, Walter SD, Russell DJ, Rosenbaum PL, Gemus M, Galuppi BE, Cunningham L (2001) 'Gross motor function of children with Down syndrome: Creation of motor growth curves.' *Archives of Physical Medicine and Rehabilatation*, **82**, 494–500.

Piper MC, Darrah J (1994) *Motor Assessment of the Developing Infant*. Philadelphia: WB Saunders.

Rasch G (1960) *Probabilistic Models for Some Intelligence and Attainment Tests*. Copenhagen: Nielson & Lydiche.

Rosenbaum P, Russell D, Cadman D, Gowland C, Jarvis S, Hardy S (1990) 'Issues in measuring change in motor function in children with cerebral palsy: A special communication.' *Physical Therapy*, **70**, 125–131.

Rosenbaum PL, Walter SD, Hanna SE, Palisano RJ, Russell DJ, Raina P, Wood E, Bartlett DJ, Galuppi BE (2002) 'Prognosis for gross motor function in cerebral palsy: Creation of motor development curves.' *Journal of the American Medical Association (in press)*.

Rosier MJ, Bishop J, Nolan T, Robertson CF, Carlin JB, Phelan PD (1994) 'Measurement of functional severity of asthma in children.' *American Journal of Critical Care Medicine*, **49**, 1434–1441.

Ruck-Gibis J, Plotkin H, Hanley J, Wood-Dauphine S (2001) 'Reliability of the Gross Motor Function Measure for children with osteogenesis imperfecta.' *Physiotherapy Canada*, **53** (1), S16.

Russell D, Rosenbaum P, Cadman D, Gowland C, Hardy S, Jarvis S (1989) 'The Gross Motor Function Measure: a means to evaluate the effects of physical therapy.' *Developmental Medicine and Child Neurology*, **31**, 341–352.

Russell DJ, Rosenbaum PL, Lane M, Gowland C, Goldsmith CH, Boyce WF, Plews N (1994) 'Training users in the Gross Motor Function Measure: Methodological and practical issues.' *Physical Therapy*, **74**, 630–636.

Russell D, Palisano R, Walter S, Rosenbaum P, Gemus M, Gowland C, Galuppi B, Lane M (1998) 'Evaluating motor function in children with Down syndrome: validity of the GMFM.' *Developmental Medicine and Child Neurology*, **40**, 693–701.

Russell DJ, Avery LM, Rosenbaum PL, Raina PS, Walter SD, Palisano RJ (2000) 'Improved scaling of the Gross Motor Function Measure for children with cerebral palsy: Evidence of reliability and validity.' *Physical Therapy*, **80**, 873–885.

Sacco D, Tylkowski C, Warf B (2000) 'Nonselective partial dorsal rhizotomy: A clinical experience with 1 year follow-up.' *Pediatric Neurosurgery*, **32**, 114–118.

Salokorpi T, Blomstedt G, Merikanto J, Jaakkola R, Sainio K, Von Wendt L (1997) 'Experiences with selective dorsal rhizotomy in Finland 1991 to 1996.' *Developmental Medicine and Child Neurology*, **39**, Suppl. 75, 30–31.

151

Schindl M, Forstner C, Kern H, Hesse S (2000) 'Treadmill training with partial body weight support in non-ambulatory patients with cerebral palsy.' *Archives of Physical Medicine and Rehabilitation*, **81**, 301–306.

Scrutton D, Rosenbaum PL (1997) 'The locomotor development of children with cerebral palsy.' *In:* Connolly KJ, Forssberg H (eds.) *Neurophysiology and Neuropsychology of Motor Development. Clinics in Developmental Medicine No. 143/144*. London: Mac Keith Press, pp 101–123.

Shrout P, Fleiss J (1979) 'Intraclass correlations: Uses in assessing rater reliability.' *Psychological Bulletin*, **86**, 420–428.

Smith R (1982) *Applications of Rasch Measurement*. Chicago: MESA Press.

Smith R (1996) 'Person fit in the Rasch model.' *Educational and Psychological Measurement*, **46**, 359–373.

Smith RM, Schumacker RE, Bush MJ (1998) 'Using item mean squares to evaluate fit to the Rasch model.' *Journal of Outcome Measurement*, **2**, 66–78.

Steel KO, Glover JE, Spasoff RA (1991) 'The Motor Control Assessment: An instrument to measure motor control in physically disabled children.' *Archives of Physical Medicine and Rehabilitation*, **72**, 549–553.

Steinbok P, Reiner A, Beauchamp R, Armstrong R, Cochrane D (1997a) 'A randomized clinical trial to compare selective dorsal rhizotomy plus physiotherapy with physiotherapy alone in children with spastic diplegic cerebral palsy.' *Developmental Medicine and Child Neurology*, **39**, 178–184

Steinbok P, Reiner A, Kestle J (1997b) 'Therapeutic electrical stimulation following selective dorsal rhizotomy in children with spastic diplegic cerebral palsy: A randomized clinical trial.' *Developmental Medicine and Child Neurology*, **39**, 515–520.

Stratford PW, Binkley JM, Riddle DL (1996) 'Health status measures: Strategies and analytic methods for assessing change scores.' *Physical Therapy*, **76**, 1109–1123.

Streiner DL, Norman GR (1989) *Health Measurement Scales: A Practical Guide to Their Development and Use*. Oxford: Oxford University Press.

Ubhi T, Bahakta B, Ives H, Allgar V, Roussounis S (2000) 'Randomized double blind placebo controlled trial of the effect of Botulinum toxin on walking in cerebral palsy.' *Archives of Disease in Childhood*, **83**, 481–487.

Van der Linden JW, Hambleton RK (eds) (1997) *Handbook of Item Response Theory*. New York: Springer.

Vohr BR, Wright LL, Dusick AM, Mele L, Verter J, Steichen JJ, Simon NP, Wilson DC, Broyles S, Bauer CR, Delaney-Black V, Yolton KA, Fleisher BE, Papile LA, Kaplan MD (2000) 'Neurodevelopmental and functional outcomes of extremely low birth weight infants in the National Institute of Child Health and Human Development Neonatal Research Network, 1993–1994.' *Pediatrics*, **105**, 1216–1226.

WeeFIM (2000) *WeeFIM System^{SM} Clinical Guide: Version 5.01*. Buffalo, NY: University at Buffalo.

Whiteneck GG, Charlifue SW, Gerhart KA, Overholser JD, Richardson GN (1992) 'Quantifying handicap: A new measure of long-term rehabilitation outcomes.' *Archives of Physical Medicine and Rehabilitation*, **73**, 519–526.

WHO (2001) *International Classification of Functioning, Disability and Health. Final Draft*. Geneva: World Health Organization.

Wood E, Rosenbaum P (2000) 'The Gross Motor Function Classification System for cerebral palsy: a study of reliability and stability over time.' *Developmental Medicine and Child Neurology*, **42**, 292–296.

Wright B, Masters G (1982) *Rating Scale Analysis*. Chicago: Mesa Press.

Wright M, Halton J, Matrin R, Barr R (1998) 'Long-term gross motor performance following treatment for acute lymphoblastic leukemia.' *Medical and Pediatric Oncology*, **31**, 86–90.

Wright T, Nicholson J (1973) 'Physiotherapy for the spastic child: an evaluation.' *Developmental Medicine and Child Neurology*, **15**, 146–163.

Wright V, Belbin G, Slack M, Jutai J, Bortolussi J, McKeever P (1997) 'A pilot evaluation of the David Hart Walker Orthosis (DHWO): a new assistive device for children with cerebral palsy (CP).' *Developmental Medicine and Child Neurology*, **39**, Suppl. 75, 35 (abstract).

Wright V, Sheil E, Drake J, Wedge J (1998) 'Evaluation of selective dorsal rhizotomy for the reduction of spasticity in cerebral palsy: a randomized controlled trial.' *Developmental Medicine and Child Neurology*, **40**, 239–247.

Young NL, Williams JI, Yoshida KK, Wright JG (2000) 'Measurement properties of the Activities Scale for Kids.' *Journal of Clinical Epidemiology*, **53**, 125–137.

GLOSSARY OF TERMS

ASCII file. A file that contains only those characters in the American Standard Code for Information Interchange (ASCII) set. These are text-only files that do not contain any of the formatting typically found in word processing, spreadsheet or database documents.

Confidence interval. The interval within which you may be reasonably confident that a measurement lies. Typically, intervals of 95% confidence are used.

Criterion testing. See "GMFM criterion testing".

Expected score. A mathematical term arrived at by summing the products of the probability of achieving a score and its value over all possible scores. The expected score is the theoretical mean score on an item for a large group of children of the same ability. (For more information see Appendix 6.)

Fisher Z transformation. A statistical tool used to normalize distributions of sample correlations so that comparisons of these correlations may be made.

GMAE. The Gross Motor Ability Estimator, a computer program used to analyse scores on the GMFM-66.

GMFM criterion testing. A test was developed to assess a person's ability to score a sample of GMFM items demonstrated on videotape. The tape contained a spectrum of items (1 through 88) and the spectrum of scores (0 through 3). A person's score was compared against an expert's score of the same videotape to determine agreement using a weighted kappa statistic. This is no longer available and GMFM users will need to assess their own reliability.

GMFM-66. An update of the GMFM-88 that includes only those 66 items identified as contributing to the measure of gross motor function in children with cerebral palsy. This new measure evaluates children using an interval score of gross motor function as opposed to the ordinal scaling of the GMFM-88.

GMFM-88. An 88-item measure designed to evaluate change in gross motor function.

Goodness of fit statistics. Statistics provided by the Rasch analysis program, which identify children (Person fit) or items (Item fit) that do not conform to the Rasch model.

Infit. A statistic that describes how well an item measures the latent trait being studied for people who function around the difficulty of the item. In the case of the GMFM this statistic describes how well an item assesses the gross motor function of children whose abilities are near to the difficulty of the item.

Interquartile range. The range within which the middle half of the sample is located. The range between the 25th and 75th percentiles of a distribution.

Interval. Pertaining to measurement that is ordered and evenly spaced, as in a ruler.

Intraclass correlation coefficient (ICC). A method to measure the effect of an uncontrolled variable among different groups in a population. An ICC is derived from an analysis of variance and allows different variance components to be identified.

Item map. A plot of the items within a measure that shows the relationship between total score on a test and the difficulty of items within that test.

Item response theory (IRT). The branch of measurement theory concerned with objective and interval-level measurement.

Item step. The difference in ability required to succeed on the next-highest response option in an item. For example, the first item step in the GMFM is the "step'" from scoring a 0 to scoring a 1.

Latent trait. That which a test attempts to measure. In the case of the GMFM the latent trait to be measured is gross motor function.

Likelihood threshold. A more general case of the Thurstone threshold indicating the ability at which a child has a specified probability of achieving at least the score of interest. For example, the 90% likelihood threshold for a score of 1 indicates the ability at which the child has a 90% probability of scoring at least a 1 (i.e. a 1, 2 or 3).

Logit. A measure of the probability of passing an item.

Noisy items. Items that do not contribute to the measurement of the underlying trait being studied.

Ordinal. Pertaining to measurement that is ordered but not necessarily evenly spaced, such as a scale of "none", "a little", "a lot".

Outfit. A statistic that describes how well an item can measure the latent trait for people who function far from the item difficulty (either above or below).

Partial credit model. A specific Rasch model in which no assumptions are made about the structure of the response categories within the items. That is, it is not assumed that achieving a score of 1 is easier than achieving a 2.

Rasch model. A one-parameter IRT model that provides sample-free estimates of item difficulty and test-free estimates of person ability.

Rating scale model. A specific Rasch model in which the difficulty of moving from one score to the next within an item is assumed to be consistent. For instance, the difficulty of moving from a score of 1 to 2 is the same as moving from a score of 2 to 3 for a given item.

Reliability. The accuracy with which results may be reproduced on repeat testing.

Sample free. The ability to reliably measure the difficulty of items with different samples of a population.

Score region. The ability region within which a given score is likely.

Standard error of measurement. The standard error of measurement as it pertains to estimates of person ability is a measure of the precision with which ability estimates could be determined from the original Rasch analysis sample. (For more information see Appendix 5.)

Step. See "Item step".

Test free. The ability to reliably measure an individual with different items from a test.

Thurstone thresholds. The ability required to be likely ($p \geq 0.5$) to achieve at least a given score. For example, the Thurstone threshold for a score of 2 is the ability required to have a 50% probability of scoring at least a 2 (either 2 or 3) on the item.

Underlying trait. See "Latent trait".

Unidimensional. Measuring a single attribute or quality. The GMFM-66 is unidimensional with respect to gross motor function.

Validity. The ability of a test to measure the underlying trait.

APPENDIX 1
GROSS MOTOR FUNCTION CLASSIFICATION
SYSTEM FOR CEREBRAL PALSY (GMFCS) *

Before 2nd Birthday

Level I   Infants move in and out of sitting and floor sit with both hands free to manipulate objects. Infants crawl on hands and knees, pull to stand and take steps holding on to furniture. Infants walk between 18 months and 2 years of age without the need for any assistive mobility device.

Level II   Infants maintain floor sitting but may need to use their hands for support to maintain balance. Infants creep on their stomach or crawl on hands and knees. Infants may pull to stand and take steps holding on to furniture.

Level III Infants maintain floor sitting when the low back is supported. Infants roll and creep forward on their stomachs.

Level IV   Infants have head control but trunk support is required for floor sitting. Infants can roll to supine and may roll to prone.

Level V   Physical impairments limit voluntary control of movement. Infants are unable to maintain antigravity head and trunk postures in prone and sitting. Infants require adult assistance to roll.

Between 2nd and 4th Birthdays

Level I   Children floor sit with both hands free to manipulate objects. Movements in and out of floor sitting and standing are performed without adult assistance. Children walk as the preferred method of mobility without the need for any assistive mobility device.

Level II   Children floor sit but may have difficulty with balance when both hands are free to manipulate objects. Movements in and out of sitting are performed without adult assistance. Children pull to stand on a stable surface. Children crawl on hands and knees with a reciprocal pattern, cruise holding onto furniture and walk using an assistive mobility device as preferred methods of mobility.

Level III Children maintain floor sitting often by "W-sitting" (sitting between flexed and internally rotated hips and knees) and may require adult assistance to assume sitting. Children creep on their stomach or crawl on hands and knees (often without reciprocal leg movements) as their primary method of self-mobility. Children may pull to stand on a stable surface and cruise short distances. Children may walk short distances indoors using an assistive mobility device and adult assistance for steering and turning.

*Adapted by permission from Palisano *et al.* (1997).

Level IV   Children sit on a chair but need adaptive seating for trunk control and to maximize hand function. Children move in and out of chair sitting with assistance from an adult or a stable surface to push or pull up on with their arms. Children may at best walk short distances with a walker and adult supervision but have difficulty turning and maintaining balance on uneven surfaces. Children are transported in the community. Children may achieve self-mobility using a power wheelchair.

Level V   Physical impairments restrict voluntary control of movement and the ability to maintain antigravity head and trunk postures. All areas of motor function are limited. Functional limitations in sitting and standing are not fully compensated for through the use of adaptive equipment and assistive technology. Children have no means of independent mobility and are transported. Some children achieve self-mobility using a power wheelchair with extensive adaptations.

Between 4th and 6th Birthdays

Level I   Children get into and out of, and sit in, a chair without the need for hand support. Children move from the floor and from chair sitting to standing without the need for objects for support. Children walk indoors and outdoors, and climb stairs. Emerging ability to run and jump.

Level II   Children sit in a chair with both hands free to manipulate objects. Children move from the floor to standing and from chair sitting to standing but often require a stable surface to push or pull up on with their arms. Children walk without the need for any assistive mobility device indoors and for short distances on level surfaces outdoors. Children climb stairs holding onto a railing but are unable to run or jump.

Level III   Children sit on a regular chair but may require pelvic or trunk support to maximize hand function. Children move in and out of chair sitting using a stable surface to push on or pull up with their arms. Children walk with an assistive mobility device on level surfaces and climb stairs with assistance from an adult. Children frequently are transported when travelling for long distances or outdoors on uneven terrain.

Level IV   Children sit on a chair but need adaptive seating for trunk control and to maximize hand function. Children move in and out of chair sitting with assistance from an adult or a stable surface to push or pull up on with their arms. Children may at best walk short distances with a walker and adult supervision but have difficulty turning and maintaining balance on uneven surfaces. Children are transported in the community. Children may achieve self-mobility using a power wheelchair.

Level V   Physical impairments restrict voluntary control of movement and the ability to maintain antigravity head and trunk postures. All areas of motor function are limited. Functional limitations in sitting and standing are not fully compensated for through the use of adaptive equipment and assistive technology. Children have no means of independent mobility and are transported. Some children achieve self-mobility using a power wheelchair with extensive adaptations.

Between 6th and 12th Birthdays

Level I   Children walk indoors and outdoors, and climb stairs without limitations. Children perform gross motor skills including running and jumping, but speed, balance and coordination are reduced.

Level II   Children walk indoors and outdoors, and climb stairs holding onto a railing, but experience limitations walking on uneven surfaces and inclines, and in crowds or confined spaces. Children have at best only minimal ability to perform gross motor skills such as running and jumping.

Level III Children walk indoors or outdoors on a level surface with an assistive mobility device. Children may climb stairs holding onto a railing. Depending on upper limb function, children propel a wheelchair manually or are transported when travelling for long distances or outdoors on uneven terrain.

Level IV   Children may maintain levels of function achieved before age 6 or rely more on wheeled mobility at home, at school and in the community. Children may achieve self-mobility using a power wheelchair.

Level V   Physical impairments restrict voluntary control of movement and the ability to maintain antigravity head and trunk postures. All areas of motor function are limited. Functional limitations in sitting and standing are not fully compensated for through the use of adaptive equipment and assistive technology. Children have no means of independent mobility and are transported. Some children achieve self-mobility using a power wheelchair with extensive adaptations.

Using the Gross Motor Ability Estimator

**To continue please click
on one of the links
below.**

Exit Tutorial

There are two ways to calculate the GMFM-66 scores with this program:

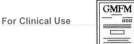

For Clinical Use

The clinical section allows you to enter data for an individual child from the GMFM score sheet. In this section you can obtain a print-out of a child's assessment information and track a child's progress over time. Information entered in this section is stored in a database so that it may be retrieved and examined at any time.

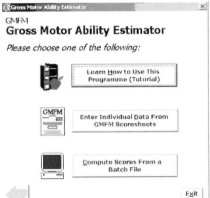

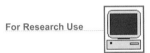

For Research Use

The research section reads in data from plain text file and outputs the GMFM-66 scores to another ASCII file. This section does not allow printouts of individual assessments, nor does it store the information for later use.

CLINICAL SECTION - Introduction

In the clinical section information about children and their GMFM assessments is stored in database files.

These files store two types of information. The **Child Information** is stored in one section of the database and contains information that only needs to be entered once for a child, such as the child's Client ID and Name.

The **Assessment Information** is stored in another part of the database and contains information that needs to be entered at each assessment, such as the date, the GMFM item scores and the name of the therapist who administered the test.

These two types of information are linked together in the database to produce **Case Summary** information that summarizes the GMFM information and plots it on a graph, allowing you to track the progress of an individual child.

Item Maps are plots that illustrate the relationship between the GMFM-66 score and the difficulties of the items in the GMFM. Both the Assessment Information and the Case Summary screens provide access to the Item Maps. More information about these maps is available later in the tutorial.

A single database file may contain information about as many or as few children as you wish. You may use the same database file for all of the children in a centre, all children in a particular program, all the children on one therapist's caseload, or maintain a separate file for each individual child.

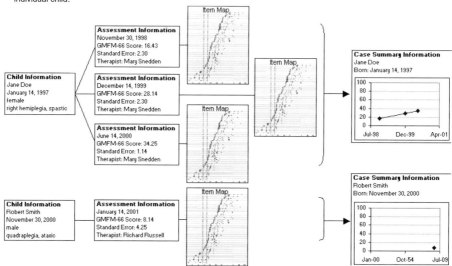

164

Step 1: Selecting a Database

The first step to entering information into the clinical section is selecting a database. If this is the first time you have used the program you will need to create a new database. Otherwise, you may open a database that you have already created.

To Create a New Database
1. Click on the [Create a New File] button.
2. Enter a name for your database.
3. Click Open.

To Open an Existing Database
1. Click on the [Open an Existing File] button.
2. Select the database file you wish to open.
3. Click Open.

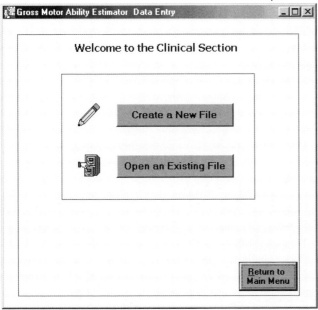

165

Step 2: Child Information Screen

Continue

Exit Tutorial

The first step to entering information into the clinical section is the Child Information screen.

Information entered here is information that only needs to be entered once - such as the child's name, date of birth and gender.

The only information that **must** be entered on this screen is the Client ID. This should be an identifier that is unique to the child and doesn't change.

Once all the information is entered for the child you can move to the next screen by clicking on one of the green arrows.

Client ID (required)
The Client ID is any combination of letters and numbers that uniquely identifies the child. The maximum length of the Client ID is 25 characters.

First Name, Last Name
The child's first name and last name are not required. If entered, they must be less than 25 characters each.

Date of Birth
The child's birthday is not required, but if omitted the child's age at assessment time will not be properly calculated. The date may be entered by selecting a date from the drop-down calendar OR by clicking on the Year, Date and Month fields and using the cursor keys.

Type of Cerebral Palsy
The diagnosis of spastic, ataxic, etc. that has been given by the developmental pediatrician, pediatric neurologist or other physician

Distribution
The area(s) of the child's body affected by cerebral palsy.

Number of Assessments

This field is read-only. It indicates the number of GMFM assessments stored in the database for the child.

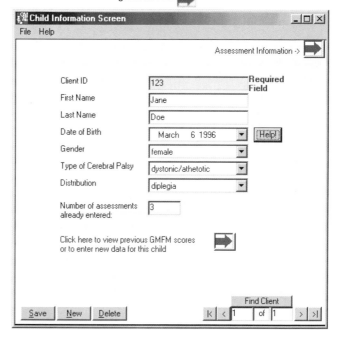

Find Client
This function allows you to search for a specific child using the criteria of either Name or Client ID.

Scrolling Buttons
The scrolling buttons beneath the Find Client button allow you to move through all the children in the current file.

More information about the buttons on the screen.

Finding a client

Return To Tutorial

To find a client that you have already entered into the database:

1. In the Search By box select one of the three methods of searching the database. You may search for clients either by their First or Last Name or, by their Client ID.
2. In the second box, beneath 'For the following name or client ID' enter the name or the client ID of the child you wish to find.
3. Click Search.
4. In the Search Results section there is a box labelled 'Name/ID': this is a drop-down box that will list all the children matching your search criteria. From this list choose the child you are searching for.
5. The remaining details for the child (date of birth, gender, etc.) will be displayed. If this is the correct child, click Select.
6. If this is not the correct child (perhaps there are two children with the same name) then select another child from the 'Name/ID' box.
7. Once you have located the child you are looking for, click Select. If you wish to cancel your search, click Cancel.

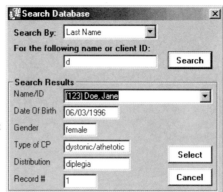

Child Information Screen buttons

Return To Tutorial

Save	Save any updated information to the database.
New	Add a new child to the database file.
Delete	Remove the child (including all assessments) from the database file.
K	Move to the first child in the database.
<	Move to the previous child in the database.
>	Move to the next child in the database.
>I	Move to the last child in the database.

Entering Birthdays and Assessment Dates

Close This Window

To quickly enter dates:
Click on the part of the date you want to change (year, month or day)

Use the up/down cursor keys on your keyboard to change your selection.
OR
Enter the day/month/year directly using the numbers on the keyboard.

To move through the day, month and year use the left/right cursor keys.

Step 3: Assessment Information Screen

The second step in the clinical section is the Assessment Information: this is where the GMFM item scores are entered and the GMFM-66 score is computed. The date of the assessment, assessing therapist, GMFCS level and the GMFM items scores are entered on this screen.

Item scores of '0', '1', '2', '3' are allowed. For items that are Not tested (NT) a 'blank' or a score of '9' can be entered and the program will treat this as missing information.

Once assessment information has been entered for a child you may view the Item Map(s) by selecting one of the options from the Item Map menu on the top of the screen.

To enter another assessment for the child click on the New button at the bottom of the screen.

Once all the assessments have been entered for the child you can move to the Case Summary screen by clicking on the forward arrow at the top-right corner of the screen.

If you made a mistake entering the child information you can return to the Child Information screen by clicking on the back arrow and the top-right corner of the screen.

The scrolling buttons at the bottom right of the screen allow you to scroll through all the assessments that have been entered for the current child. To scroll through assessments for a different child you must first go back to the Child Information screen and select another child.

|< < 1 of 3 > >|

Assessment Date
The date on which the GMFM was administered to the child.

Therapist
The name or ID of the therapist who administered the GMFM.

GMFCS Level
The Gross Motor Function Classification System level to which the child belongs.

More Information on the GMFCS

Use GMFM-66 Scores Only
Check this box to automatically skip down the list to each of the 66 items of the GMFM-66. Uncheck this box if you wish to enter all 88 GMFM items.

Auto Scroll through items
Check this box if you wish to automatically jump to the next item once a valid item score has been entered. If this box is unchecked then you must manually move to the next item using either the Cursor Down or Enter keys on the keyboard.

Please Note:
Screen may appear differently depending on screen resolution.

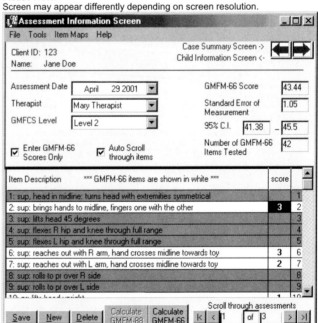

More information about the buttons on the screen

Gross Motor Function Classification System (GMFCS)

Continue

Exit Tutorial

Before 2nd Birthday

Level 1   Infants move in and out of sitting and floor sit with both hands free to manipulate objects. Infants crawl on hands and knees, pull to stand and take steps holding on to furniture. Infants walk between 18 months and 2 years of age without the need for any assistive mobility device.

Level 2   Infants maintain floor sitting but may need to use their hands for support to maintain balance. Infants creep on their stomach or crawl on hands and knees. Infants may pull to stand and take steps holding on to furniture.

Level 3   Infants maintain floor sitting when the low back is supported. Infants roll and creep forward on their stomachs.

Level 4   Infants have head control but trunk support is required for floor sitting. Infants can roll to supine and may roll to prone.

Level 5   Physical impairments limit voluntary control of movement. Infants are unable to maintain antigravity head and trunk postures in prone and sitting. Infants require adult assistance to roll.

Between 2nd and 4th Birthday

Level 1   Children floor sit with both hands free to manipulate objects. Movements in and out of floor sitting and standing are performed without adult assistance. Children walk as the preferred method of mobility without the need for any assistive mobility device.

Level 2   Children floor sit but may have difficulty with balance when both hands are free to manipulate objects. Movements in and out of sitting are performed without adult assistance. Children pull to stand on a stable surface. Children crawl on hands and knees with a reciprocal pattern, cruise holding onto furniture and walk using an assistive mobility device as preferred methods of mobility.

Level 3   Children maintain floor sitting often by "W-sitting" (sitting between flexed and internally rotated hips and knees) and may require adult assistance to assume sitting. Children creep on their stomach or crawl on hands and knees (often without reciprocal leg movements) as their primary method of self-mobility. Children may pull to stand on a stable surface and cruise short distances. Children may walk short distances indoors using an assistive mobility device and adult assistance for steering and turning.

Level 4   Children sit on a chair but need adaptive seating for trunk control and to maximize hand function. Children move in and out of chair sitting with assistance from an adult or a stable surface to push or pull up on with their arms. Children may at best walk short distances with a walker and adult supervision but have difficulty turning and maintaining balance on uneven surfaces. Children are transported in the community. Children may achieve self-mobility using a power wheelchair.

Level 5   Physical impairments restrict voluntary control of movement and the ability to maintain antigravity head and trunk postures. All areas of motor function are limited. Functional limitations in sitting and standing are not fully compensated for through the use of adaptive equipment and assistive technology. Children have no means of independent mobility and are transported. Some children achieve self-mobility using a power wheelchair with extensive adaptations.

Between 4th and 6th Birthday

Level 1   Children get into and out of, and sit in, a chair without the need for hand support. Children move from the floor and from chair sitting to standing without the need for objects for support. Children walk indoors and outdoors, and climb stairs. Emerging ability to run and jump.

Level 2   Children sit in a chair with both hands free to manipulate objects. Children move from the floor to standing and from chair sitting to standing but often require a stable surface to push or pull up on with their arms. Children walk without the need for any assistive mobility device indoors and for short distances on level surfaces outdoors. Children climb stairs holding onto a railing but are unable to run or jump.

Level 3   Children sit on a regular chair but may require pelvic or trunk support to maximize hand function. Children move in and out of chair sitting using a stable surface to push on or pull up with their arms. Children walk with an assistive mobility device on level surfaces and climb stairs with assistance from an adult. Children frequently are transported when travelling for long distances or outdoors on uneven terrain.

Level 4   Children sit on a chair but need adaptive seating for trunk control and to maximize hand function. Children move in and out of chair sitting with assistance from an adult or a stable surface to push or pull up on with their arms. Children may at best walk short distances with a walker and adult supervision but have difficulty turning and maintaining balance on uneven surfaces. Children are transported in the community. Children may achieve self-mobility using a power wheelchair.

Level 5   Physical impairments restrict voluntary control of movement and the ability to maintain antigravity head and trunk postures. All areas of motor function are limited. Functional limitations in sitting and standing are not fully compensated for through the use of adaptive equipment and assistive technology. Children have no means of independent mobility and are transported. Some children achieve self-mobility using a power wheelchair with extensive adaptations.

Between 6th and 12th Birthday

Level 1   Children walk indoors and outdoors, and climb stairs without limitations. Children perform gross motor skills including running and jumping, but speed, balance and coordination are reduced.

Level 2   Children walk indoors and outdoors, and climb stairs holding onto a railing, but experience limitations walking on uneven surfaces and inclines, and in crowds or confined spaces. Children have at best only minimal ability to perform gross motor skills such as running and jumping.

Level 3   Children walk indoors or outdoors on a level surface with an assistive mobility device. Children may climb stairs holding onto a railing. Depending on upper limb function, children propel a wheelchair manually or are transported when travelling for long distances or outdoors on uneven terrain.

Level 4   Children may maintain levels of function achieved before age 6 or rely more on wheeled mobility at home, at school, and in the community. Children may achieve self-mobility using a power wheelchair.

Level 5   Physical impairments restrict voluntary control of movement and the ability to maintain antigravity head and trunk postures. All areas of motor function are limited. Functional limitations in sitting and standing are not fully compensated for through the use of adaptive equipment and assistive technology. Children have no means of independent mobility and are transported. Some children achieve self-mobility using a power wheelchair with extensive adaptations.

RESEARCH SECTION - Overview

In the research section information for a number of children is input in the form of an ASCII text file. This 'batch' file is read into the program and another batch file containing the GMFM-66 scores for each child is output.

This section is intended for studies or centres where the GMFM item scores have already been entered into a statistical or database package and the user wishes to calculate the GMFM-66 scores without re-entering the GMFM assessments for each child.

This section assumes that the user has previous experience with database programmes and/or statistical packages and is capable of converting existing data into text format.

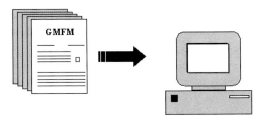

175

Step 1: Formatting the input file

Use the following guidelines to format a batch file:

1. The data must be in simple text format. Codes such as those created by Word, WordPerfect and WordPro are not allowed. The Notepad utility creates acceptable formats.

2. Each child's scores must be entered on a separate line in the batch file and must contain an identifier followed by the item scores in order.

3. The identifier is likely to be the child's client ID but may be any alpha-numeric code up to 25 characters.

4. You may choose between entering all 88 items (the 66 GMFM-66 items. However, a score must be entered for every item (88 or 66 respectively) and r scores should be represented by a space or a '9'.

5. Only the Client ID and the GMFM items are acce by the program, all other fields must be removed.

6. All entries in the file must contain the same num items - i.e. all GMFM-66 scores or all GMFM-88 sc but not a combination of the two.

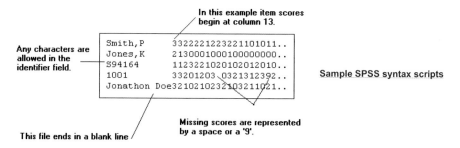

In this example item scores begin at column 13.

```
Smith,P      3322221223221101011..
Jones,K      2130001000100000000..
S94164       1123321020102012010..
1001         33201203 0321312392..
Jonathon Doe32102102321 03211021..
```

Any characters are allowed in the identifier field.

This file ends in a blank line

Missing scores are represented by a space or a '9'.

Sample SPSS syntax scripts

SPSS Syntax Samples

Return To Tutorial

The following examples can be run in SPSS to produce ASCII files that meet the criteria of the GMAE. These examples assume that there is a field entitled ClientID that contains client identifiers of no more than 25 characters in length and that the scores for the items in the GMFM are entered into fields labelled GMFM_1 through to GMFM_88.

Sample syntax file to export all 88 items from the GMFM:
```
WRITE OUTFILE = "C:\WINDOWS\Desktop\Batch_File.ASC"
/STUDYID *
GMFM_1 TO GMFM_88 (88(F1)).
EXECUTE.
```

Sample syntax file if only the GMFM-66 items have been entered:
```
WRITE OUTFILE = "C:\WINDOWS\Desktop\Batch_File.ASC"
/STUDYID *
GMFM_1 TO GMFM_66 (66(F1)).
EXECUTE.
```

Step 2: Specifying file details

To calculate GMFM-66 scores from your batch file you must first provide some information about the format of the file.

1. If all 88 GMFM items are entered into the batch file then leave the first option selected. If only the 66 GMFM-66 items are contained in the batch file then click on the second option.

2. Enter the number of the column at which the item scores begin. Note that the item scores must begin at the same column for all children in the file. This column number will generally be one larger than the longest Client ID in the batch file.

3. Click on Select Data File to specify which batch files to calculate the scores from.

4. Click on Select Output File to specify the name and location of the file where you would like the scores to be written. You may create a new file.

5. Click on the forward arrow.

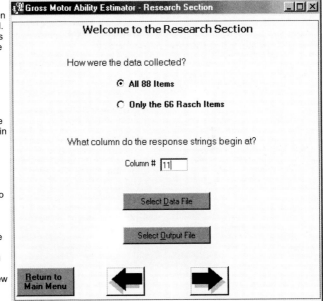

Step 3: Verify the file details

Read over the details listed on this screen and if everything is correct click the forward arrow to calculate the scores.

To change any of the details click on the back arrow to return to the previous screen.

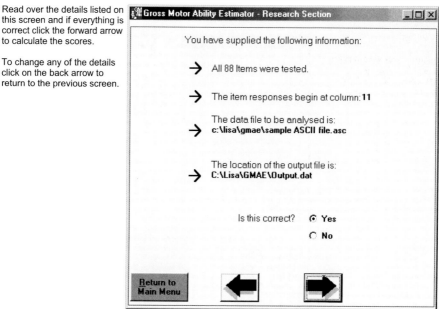

Step 4: View the GMFM-66 scores

Finish Tutorial

Once the calculation of all of the GMFM-66 scores is complete they will appear on-screen. These scores are also written to the output file you specified.

Information is written to the output file in comma separated values (CSV) format.

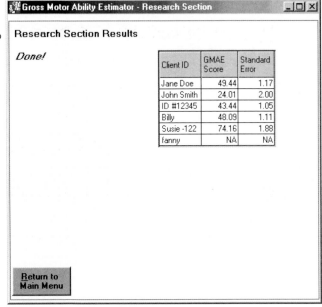

Gross Motor Ability Estimator - Research Section

Research Section Results

Done!

Client ID	GMAE Score	Standard Error
Jane Doe	49.44	1.17
John Smith	24.01	2.00
ID #12345	43.44	1.05
Billy	48.09	1.11
Susie -122	74.16	1.88
fanny	NA	NA

Return to Main Menu

179

APPENDIX 3
SCORING THE GMFM-88 AND GMFM-66: CASE SCENARIO OF SUSIE

This appendix demonstrates the method of scoring for the GMFM-66 and GMFM-88, using as our example the case of Susie, aged 20 months at her first assessment in 1989, who had cerebral palsy classified at that time as moderate.

The first two figures reproduce her score sheets at the initial and six-month follow-up assessments. The data from these has been entered into the GMAE program, producing item maps by difficulty order and by item order for each assessment, shown as Figures A3.3–A3.4 and A3.5–A3.6 respectively, and a case summary report (Fig. A3.7) detailing the change score between the two assessments.

Finally, Figure A3.8 shows how Susie's follow-up assessment would be scored using the new GMFM score sheet (2002).

GROSS MOTOR FUNCTION MEASURE
GMFM

SCORE SHEET

Child's Name: _Susie_   I.D. # : _1234_

Date of Birth: _87_ / _07_ / _07_   Assessment date: _89_ / _04_ / _03_
           yy / mm / dd   yy / mm / dd

Diagnosis: _Mixed CP_   Severity: ☐ ☑ ☐
                                                        Mild Moderate Severe

Evaluator's Name _Mary Therapist_

Testing Conditions (e.g. room, clothing, time, others present)
Physiotherapy gym - Mom present   _9:00 am._
diaper, comfortable   _Initial assessment_

The GMFM is a standardized observational instrument designed and validated to measure change in gross motor function over time in children with cerebral palsy.

| *SCORING KEY | 0 = does not initiate |
| 1 = initiates |
| 2 = partially completes |
| 3 = completes |

*Unless otherwise specified, "initiates" is defined as completion of less than 10% of the item. "Partially completes" is defined as completion of 10% to less than 100%.

The scoring key is meant to be a general guideline. However, most of the items have specific descriptors for each score. It is imperative that the **guidelines be used for scoring each item.**

Contact address:
     Dianne Russell, Gross Motor Measure Group, Chedoke-McMaster Hospitals, Chedoke Hospital, Building 74, Room 29, Box 2000, Station "A", Hamilton, Ontario L8N 3Z5

Children's Developmental Rehabilitation Programme at Chedoke-McMaster Hospitals, Hamilton, Ontario, Hugh MacMillan Rehabilitation Centre, Toronto, Ontario, and McMaster University, Hamilton, Ontario

Check (✔) the appropriate score:

Item   A: **LYING AND ROLLING**   **SCORE**

#	Item	0	1	2	3	#
1.	SUP, HEAD IN MIDLINE: TURNS HEAD WITH EXTREMITIES SYMMETRICAL				✔	1.
2.	SUP: BRINGS HANDS TO MIDLINE, FINGERS ONE WITH THE OTHER				✔	2.
3.	SUP: LIFTS HEAD 45°	✔				3.
4.	SUP: FLEXES R HIP & KNEE THROUGH FULL RANGE			✔		4.
5.	SUP: FLEXES L HIP AND KNEE THROUGH FULL RANGE			✔		5.
6.	SUP: REACHES OUT WITH R ARM, HAND CROSSES MIDLINE TOWARD TOY				✔	6.
7.	SUP: REACHES OUT WITH L ARM, HAND CROSSES MIDLINE TOWARD TOY				✔	7.
8.	SUP: ROLLS TO PR OVER R SIDE				✔	8.
9.	SUP: ROLLS TO PR OVER L SIDE			✔		9.
10.	PR: LIFTS HEAD UPRIGHT				✔	10.
11.	PR ON FOREARMS: LIFTS HEAD UPRIGHT, ELBOWS EXT., CHEST RAISED				✔	11.
12.	PR ON FOREARMS: WEIGHT ON R FOREARM, FULLY EXTENDS OPPOSITE ARM FORWARD	✔				12.
13.	PR ON FOREARMS: WEIGHT ON L FOREARM, FULLY EXTENDS OPPOSITE ARM FORWARD	✔				13.
14.	PR: ROLLS TO SUP OVER R SIDE	✔				14.
15.	PR: ROLLS TO SUP OVER L SIDE	✔				15.
16.	PR: PIVOTS TO R 90° USING EXTREMITIES				✔	16.
17.	PR: PIVOTS TO L 90° USING EXTREMITIES				✔	17.

TOTAL DIMENSION A   33

Item   B: **SITTING**   **SCORE**

#	Item	0	1	2	3	#
18.	SUP, HANDS GRASPED BY EXAMINER: PULLS SELF TO SITTING WITH HEAD CONTROL				✔	18.
19.	SUP: ROLLS TO R SIDE, ATTAINS SITTING	✔				19.
20.	SUP: ROLLS TO L SIDE, ATTAINS SITTING	✔				20.
21.	SIT ON MAT, SUPPORTED AT THORAX BY THERAPIST: LIFTS HEAD UPRIGHT, MAINTAINS 3 SECONDS	✔				21.
22.	SIT ON MAT, SUPPORTED AT THORAX BY THERAPIST: LIFTS HEAD TO MIDLINE, MAINTAINS 10 SECONDS	✔				22.
23.	SIT ON MAT, ARM(S) PROPPING: MAINTAINS, 5 SECONDS				✔	23.
24.	SIT ON MAT: MAINTAINS, ARMS FREE, 3 SECONDS				✔	24.
25.	SIT ON MAT WITH SMALL TOY IN FRONT: LEANS FORWARD, TOUCHES TOY, RE-ERECTS WITHOUT ARM PROPPING			✔		25.
26.	SIT ON MAT: TOUCHES TOY PLACED 45° BEHIND CHILD'S R SIDE, RETURNS TO START				✔	26.
27.	SIT ON MAT: TOUCHES TOY PLACED 45° BEHIND CHILD'S L SIDE, RETURNS TO START				✔	27.
28.	R SIDE SIT: MAINTAINS, ARMS FREE, 5 SECONDS			✔		28.
29.	L SIDE SIT: MAINTAINS, ARMS FREE, 5 SECONDS			✔		29.
30.	SIT ON MAT: LOWERS TO PR WITH CONTROL		✔			30.
31.	SIT ON MAT WITH FEET IN FRONT: ATTAINS 4 POINT OVER R SIDE				✔	31.
32.	SIT ON MAT WITH FEET IN FRONT: ATTAINS 4 POINT OVER L SIDE	✔				32.
33.	SIT ON MAT: PIVOTS 90°, WITHOUT ARMS ASSISTING			✔		33.
34.	SIT ON BENCH: MAINTAINS, ARMS AND FEET FREE, 10 SECONDS				✔	34.
35.	STD: ATTAINS SIT ON SMALL BENCH		✔			35.
36.	ON THE FLOOR: ATTAINS SIT ON SMALL BENCH		✔			36.
37.	ON THE FLOOR: ATTAINS SIT ON LARGE BENCH		✔			37.

TOTAL DIMENSION B   33

Item C: CRAWLING AND KNEELING · SCORE

#	Item	0	1	2	3	
38.	PR: CREEPS FORWARD 6'		✓			38.
39.	4 POINT: MAINTAINS, WEIGHT ON HANDS AND KNEES, 10 SECONDS				✓	39.
40.	4 POINT: ATTAINS SIT ARMS FREE			✓		40.
41.	PR: ATTAINS 4 POINT, WEIGHT ON HANDS AND KNEES			✓		41.
42.	4 POINT: REACHES FORWARD WITH R ARM, HAND ABOVE SHOULDER LEVEL				✓	42.
43.	4 POINT: REACHES FORWARD WITH L ARM, HAND ABOVE SHOULDER LEVEL			✓		43.
44.	4 POINT: CRAWLS OR HITCHES FORWARD 6'		✓			44.
45.	4 POINT: CRAWLS RECIPROCALLY FORWARD 6'		✓			45.
46.	4 POINT: CRAWLS UP 4 STEPS ON HANDS AND KNEES/FEET	✓				46.
47.	4 POINT: CRAWLS BACKWARDS DOWN 4 STEPS ON HANDS AND KNEES/FEET	✓				47.
48.	SIT ON MAT: ATTAINS HIGH KN USING ARMS, MAINTAINS, ARMS FREE, 10 SECONDS	✓				48.
49.	HIGH KN: ATTAINS HALF KN ON R KNEE USING ARMS, MAINTAINS, ARMS FREE, 10 SECONDS	✓				49.
50.	HIGH KN: ATTAINS HALF KN ON L KNEE USING ARMS, MAINTAINS, ARMS FREE, 10 SECONDS	✓				50.
51.	HIGH KN: KN WALKS FORWARD 10 STEPS, ARMS FREE	✓				51.

TOTAL DIMENSION C — 15

Item D: STANDING · SCORE

#	Item	0	1	2	3	
52.	ON THE FLOOR: PULLS TO STD AT LARGE BENCH		✓			52.
53.	STD: MAINTAINS, ARMS FREE, 3 SECONDS	✓				53.
54.	STD: HOLDING ON TO LARGE BENCH WITH ONE HAND, LIFTS R FOOT, 3 SECONDS	✓				54.
55.	STD: HOLDING ON TO LARGE BENCH WITH ONE HAND, LIFTS L FOOT, 3 SECONDS	✓				55.
56.	STD: MAINTAINS, ARMS FREE, 20 SECONDS	✓				56.
57.	STD: LIFTS L FOOT, ARMS FREE, 10 SECONDS	✓				57.
58.	STD: LIFTS R FOOT, ARMS FREE, 10 SECONDS	✓				58.
59.	SIT ON SMALL BENCH: ATTAINS STD WITHOUT USING ARMS	✓				59.
60.	HIGH KN: ATTAINS STD THROUGH HALF KN ON R KNEE, WITHOUT USING ARMS	✓				60.
61.	HIGH KN: ATTAINS STD THROUGH HALF KN ON L KNEE, WITHOUT USING ARMS	✓				61.
62.	STD: LOWERS TO SIT ON FLOOR WITH CONTROL, ARMS FREE	✓				62.
63.	STD: ATTAINS SQUAT, ARMS FREE	✓				63.
64.	STD: PICKS UP OBJECT FROM FLOOR, ARMS FREE, RETURNS TO STAND	✓				64.

TOTAL DIMENSION D — 1

183

Item	E. WALKING, RUNNING AND JUMPING	SCORE				
65.	STD, 2 HANDS ON LARGE BENCH: CRUISES 5 STEPS TO R	0 ☑	1 ☐	2 ☐	3 ☐	65.
66.	STD, 2 HANDS ON LARGE BENCH: CRUISES 5 STEPS TO L	0 ☑	1 ☐	2 ☐	3 ☐	66.
67.	STD, 2 HANDS HELD: WALKS FORWARD 10 STEPS	0 ☑	1 ☐	2 ☐	3 ☐	67.
68.	STD, 1 HAND HELD: WALKS FORWARD 10 STEPS	0 ☑	1 ☐	2 ☐	3 ☐	68.
69.	STD: WALKS FORWARD 10 STEPS	0 ☑	1 ☐	2 ☐	3 ☐	69.
70.	STD: WALKS FORWARD 10 STEPS, STOPS, TURNS 180°, RETURNS	0 ☑	1 ☐	2 ☐	3 ☐	70.
71.	STD: WALKS BACKWARD 10 STEPS	0 ☑	1 ☐	2 ☐	3 ☐	71.
72.	STD: WALKS FORWARD 10 STEPS, CARRYING A LARGE OBJECT WITH 2 HANDS	0 ☑	1 ☐	2 ☐	3 ☐	72.
73.	STD: WALKS FORWARD 10 CONSECUTIVE STEPS BETWEEN PARALLEL LINES 8" APART	0 ☑	1 ☐	2 ☐	3 ☐	73.
74.	STD: WALKS FORWARD 10 CONSECUTIVE STEPS ON A STRAIGHT LINE ¾" WIDE	0 ☑	1 ☐	2 ☐	3 ☐	74.
75.	STD: STEPS OVER STICK AT KNEE LEVEL, R FOOT LEADING	0 ☑	1 ☐	2 ☐	3 ☐	75.
76.	STD: STEPS OVER STICK AT KNEE LEVEL, L FOOT LEADING	0 ☑	1 ☐	2 ☐	3 ☐	76.
77.	STD: RUNS 15 FEET, STOPS & RETURNS	0 ☑	1 ☐	2 ☐	3 ☐	77.
78.	STD: KICKS BALL WITH R FOOT	0 ☑	1 ☐	2 ☐	3 ☐	78.
79.	STD: KICKS BALL WITH L FOOT	0 ☑	1 ☐	2 ☐	3 ☐	79.
80.	STD: JUMPS 12" HIGH, BOTH FEET SIMULTANEOUSLY	0 ☑	1 ☐	2 ☐	3 ☐	80.
81.	STD: JUMPS FORWARD 12", BOTH FEET SIMULTANEOUSLY	0 ☑	1 ☐	2 ☐	3 ☐	81.
82.	STD ON R FOOT: HOPS ON R FOOT 10 TIMES WITHIN A 24" CIRCLE	0 ☑	1 ☐	2 ☐	3 ☐	82.
83.	STD ON L FOOT: HOPS ON L FOOT 10 TIMES WITHIN A 24" CIRCLE	0 ☑	1 ☐	2 ☐	3 ☐	83.
84.	STD, HOLDING 1 RAIL: WALKS UP 4 STEPS, HOLDING 1 RAIL, ALTERNATING FEET	0 ☑	1 ☐	2 ☐	3 ☐	84.
85.	STD, HOLDING 1 RAIL: WALKS DOWN 4 STEPS, HOLDING 1 RAIL, ALTERNATING FEET	0 ☑	1 ☐	2 ☐	3 ☐	85.
86.	STD: WALKS UP 4 STEPS, ALTERNATING FEET	0 ☑	1 ☐	2 ☐	3 ☐	86.
87.	STD: WALKS DOWN 4 STEPS, ALTERNATING FEET	0 ☑	1 ☐	2 ☐	3 ☐	87.
88.	STD ON 6" STEP: JUMPS OFF, BOTH FEET SIMULTANEOUSLY	0 ☑	1 ☐	2 ☐	3 ☐	88.

TOTAL DIMENSION E [*0*]

Was this assessment indicative of this child's "regular" performance?   YES ☑ NO ☐

COMMENTS:

Refused items   12-15, 22, 21, 46, 47

GMFM

SUMMARY SCORE

DIMENSION	CALCULATION OF DIMENSION % SCORES	GOAL AREA (indicated with ✓ check)
A. Lying & Rolling	$\dfrac{\text{Total Dimension A}}{51} = \dfrac{33}{51} \times 100 = \underline{65}$ %	A. ☐
B. Sitting	$\dfrac{\text{Total Dimension B}}{60} = \dfrac{33}{60} \times 100 = \underline{55}$ %	B. ☑
C. Crawling & Kneeling	$\dfrac{\text{Total Dimension C}}{42} = \dfrac{15}{42} \times 100 = \underline{36}$ %	C. ☑
D. Standing	$\dfrac{\text{Total Dimension D}}{39} = \dfrac{1}{39} \times 100 = \underline{3}$ %	D. ☑
E. Walking, Running & Jumping	$\dfrac{\text{Total Dimension E}}{72} = \dfrac{0}{72} \times 100 = \underline{0}$ %	E. ☐

TOTAL SCORE $= \dfrac{\text{\% A + \% B + \% C + \% D + \% E}}{\text{Total \# of Dimensions}}$

$= \dfrac{65 + 55 + 36 + 3 + 0}{5} = \dfrac{159}{5} = \underline{32}$ %

GOAL TOTAL SCORE $= \dfrac{\text{Sum of \% scores for each dimension identified as a goal area}}{\text{\# Goal areas}}$

$= \dfrac{55 + 36 + 3}{3} = \underline{31}$ %

185

TESTING WITH AIDS/ORTHOSES

Indicate below with a check (✓) which aid/orthosis was used and what dimension it was first applied. (There may be more than one).

Aid	Dimension	Orthosis	Dimension
Rollator/pusher............................ ☐	_____	Hip Control................................ ☐	_____
Walker... ☐	_____	Knee Control.............................. ☐	_____
H Frame crutches........................ ☐	_____	Ankle-foot Control...................... ☐	_____
Crutches...................................... ☐	_____	Foot Control............................... ☐	_____
Quad Cane................................... ☐	_____	Shoes.. ☐	
Cane... ☐	_____	None.. ☑	
None... ☑	_____	Other _____ ☐	_____
Other _____ ☐	_____	(please specify)	
(please specify)			

SUMMARY SCORE USING AIDS/ORTHOSES

DIMENSION	CALCULATION OF DIMENSION % SCORES	GOAL AREA (indicated with ✓ check)
A. Lying & Rolling	$\dfrac{\text{Total Dimension A}}{51}$ = $\dfrac{\quad}{51}$ x 100 = _____ %	A. ☐
B. Sitting	$\dfrac{\text{Total Dimension B}}{60}$ = $\dfrac{\quad}{60}$ x 100 = _____ %	B. ☐
C. Crawling & Kneeling	$\dfrac{\text{Total Dimension C}}{42}$ = $\dfrac{\quad}{42}$ x 100 = _____ %	C. ☐
D. Standing	$\dfrac{\text{Total Dimension D}}{39}$ = $\dfrac{\quad}{39}$ x 100 = _____ %	D. ☐
E. Walking, Running & Jumping	$\dfrac{\text{Total Dimension E}}{72}$ = $\dfrac{\quad}{72}$ x 100 = _____ %	E. ☐

TOTAL SCORE = $\dfrac{\text{\% A + \% B + \% C + \% D + \% E}}{\text{Total \# of Dimensions}}$

= $\dfrac{\quad + \quad + \quad + \quad + \quad}{5}$ = $\dfrac{\quad}{5}$ = _____ %

GOAL TOTAL SCORE = $\dfrac{\text{Sum of \% scores for each dimension identified as a goal area}}{\text{\# Goal areas}}$

= _____ = ___ %

GROSS MOTOR FUNCTION MEASURE
GMFM

SCORE SHEET

Child's Name: _Susie_   I.D. #: _1234_

Date of Birth: _87_/_07_/_07_   Assessment date: _89_/_10_/_06_
              yy / mm / dd   yy / mm / dd

Diagnosis: _Mixed CP_   Severity: ☐ ☑ ☐
                                                  Mild Moderate Severe

Evaluator's Name _Mary Therapist_

Testing Conditions (e.g. room, clothing, time, others present)

Physiotherapy gym – 9:30 am

Mother present

diaper only   _Repeat Assessment_

The GMFM is a standardized observational instrument designed and validated to measure change in gross motor function over time in children with cerebral palsy.

> *SCORING KEY   0 = does not initiate
>   1 = initiates
>   2 = partially completes
>   3 = completes

*Unless otherwise specified, "initiates" is defined as completion of less than 10% of the item. "Partially completes" is defined as completion of 10% to less than 100%.

The scoring key is meant to be a general guideline. However, most of the items have specific descriptors for each score. It is imperative that the **guidelines be used for scoring each item.**

Contact address:
    Dianne Russell, Gross Motor Measure Group, Chedoke-McMaster Hospitals, Chedoke Hospital, Building 74, Room 29, Box 2000, Station "A", Hamilton, Ontario L8N 3Z5

Children's Developmental Rehabilitation Programme at Chedoke-McMaster Hospitals, Hamilton, Ontario, Hugh MacMillan Rehabilitation Centre, Toronto, Ontario, and McMaster University, Hamilton, Ontario

Check (✓) the appropriate score:

Item	A: LYING AND ROLLING		SCORE			
		0	1	2	3	
1.	SUP, HEAD IN MIDLINE: TURNS HEAD WITH EXTREMITIES SYMMETRICAL	☐	☐	☐	✓	1.
2.	SUP: BRINGS HANDS TO MIDLINE, FINGERS ONE WITH THE OTHER	☐	☐	☐	✓	2.
3.	SUP: LIFTS HEAD 45°	☐	☐	✓	☐	3.
4.	SUP: FLEXES R HIP & KNEE THROUGH FULL RANGE	☐	☐	✓	☐	4.
5.	SUP: FLEXES L HIP AND KNEE THROUGH FULL RANGE	☐	☐	✓	☐	5.
6.	SUP: REACHES OUT WITH R ARM, HAND CROSSES MIDLINE TOWARD TOY	☐	☐	☐	✓	6.
7.	SUP: REACHES OUT WITH L ARM, HAND CROSSES MIDLINE TOWARD TOY	☐	☐	☐	✓	7.
8.	SUP: ROLLS TO PR OVER R SIDE	☐	☐	☐	✓	8.
9.	SUP: ROLLS TO PR OVER L SIDE	☐	☐	☐	✓	9.
10.	PR: LIFTS HEAD UPRIGHT	☐	☐	☐	✓	10.
11.	PR ON FOREARMS: LIFTS HEAD UPRIGHT, ELBOWS EXT., CHEST RAISED	☐	☐	☐	✓	11.
12.	PR ON FOREARMS: WEIGHT ON R FOREARM, FULLY EXTENDS OPPOSITE ARM FORWARD	☐	☐	✓	☐	12.
13.	PR ON FOREARMS: WEIGHT ON L FOREARM, FULLY EXTENDS OPPOSITE ARM FORWARD	☐	☐	✓	☐	13.
14.	PR: ROLLS TO SUP OVER R SIDE	✓	☐	☐	☐	14.
15.	PR: ROLLS TO SUP OVER L SIDE	✓	☐	☐	☐	15.
16.	PR: PIVOTS TO R 90° USING EXTREMITIES	☐	☐	☐	✓	16.
17.	PR: PIVOTS TO L 90° USING EXTREMITIES	✓	☐	☐	☐	17.

TOTAL DIMENSION A 　　37

Item	B: SITTING		SCORE			
		0	1	2	3	
18.	SUP, HANDS GRASPED BY EXAMINER: PULLS SELF TO SITTING WITH HEAD CONTROL	☐	☐	☐	✓	18.
19.	SUP: ROLLS TO R SIDE, ATTAINS SITTING	✓	☐	☐	☐	19.
20.	SUP: ROLLS TO L SIDE, ATTAINS SITTING	✓	☐	☐	☐	20.
21.	SIT ON MAT, SUPPORTED AT THORAX BY THERAPIST: LIFTS HEAD UPRIGHT, MAINTAINS 3 SECONDS	☐	☐	☐	✓	21.
22.	SIT ON MAT, SUPPORTED AT THORAX BY THERAPIST: LIFTS HEAD TO MIDLINE, MAINTAINS 10 SECONDS	☐	☐	✓	☐	22.
23.	SIT ON MAT, ARM(S) PROPPING: MAINTAINS, 5 SECONDS	☐	☐	☐	✓	23.
24.	SIT ON MAT: MAINTAINS, ARMS FREE, 3 SECONDS	☐	☐	☐	✓	24.
25.	SIT ON MAT WITH SMALL TOY IN FRONT: LEANS FORWARD, TOUCHES TOY, RE-ERECTS WITHOUT ARM PROPPING	☐	☐	✓	☐	25.
26.	SIT ON MAT: TOUCHES TOY PLACED 45° BEHIND CHILD'S R SIDE, RETURNS TO START	☐	☐	☐	✓	26.
27.	SIT ON MAT: TOUCHES TOY PLACED 45° BEHIND CHILD'S L SIDE, RETURNS TO START	☐	✓	☐	☐	27.
28.	R SIDE SIT: MAINTAINS, ARMS FREE, 5 SECONDS	☐	☐	☐	✓	28.
29.	L SIDE SIT: MAINTAINS, ARMS FREE, 5 SECONDS	☐	☐	☐	✓	29.
30.	SIT ON MAT: LOWERS TO PR WITH CONTROL	✓	☐	☐	☐	30.
31.	SIT ON MAT WITH FEET IN FRONT: ATTAINS 4 POINT OVER R SIDE	✓	☐	☐	☐	31.
32.	SIT ON MAT WITH FEET IN FRONT: ATTAINS 4 POINT OVER L SIDE	☐	☐	☐	✓	32.
33.	SIT ON MAT: PIVOTS 90°, WITHOUT ARMS ASSISTING	☐	☐	✓	☐	33.
34.	SIT ON BENCH: MAINTAINS, ARMS AND FEET FREE, 10 SECONDS	☐	☐	✓	☐	34.
35.	STD: ATTAINS SIT ON SMALL BENCH	☐	☐	✓	☐	35.
36.	ON THE FLOOR: ATTAINS SIT ON SMALL BENCH	☐	☐	✓	☐	36.
37.	ON THE FLOOR: ATTAINS SIT ON LARGE BENCH	☐	☐	✓	☐	37.

TOTAL DIMENSION B 　　39

Item	C: **CRAWLING AND KNEELING**		SCORE			
38.	PR: CREEPS FORWARD 6'	0 ☑	1 ☐	2 ☐	3 ☐	38.
39.	4 POINT: MAINTAINS, WEIGHT ON HANDS AND KNEES, 10 SECONDS	0 ☐	1 ☐	2 ☐	3 ☑	39.
40.	4 POINT: ATTAINS SIT ARMS FREE	0 ☐	1 ☐	2 ☑	3 ☐	40.
41.	PR: ATTAINS 4 POINT, WEIGHT ON HANDS AND KNEES	0 ☐	1 ☐	2 ☐	3 ☑	41.
42.	4 POINT: REACHES FORWARD WITH R ARM, HAND ABOVE SHOULDER LEVEL	0 ☐	1 ☐	2 ☐	3 ☑	42.
43.	4 POINT: REACHES FORWARD WITH L ARM, HAND ABOVE SHOULDER LEVEL	0 ☐	1 ☐	2 ☐	3 ☑	43.
44.	4 POINT: CRAWLS OR HITCHES FORWARD 6'	0 ☐	1 ☐	2 ☐	3 ☑	44.
45.	4 POINT: CRAWLS RECIPROCALLY FORWARD 6'	0 ☐	1 ☐	2 ☑	3 ☐	45.
46.	4 POINT: CRAWLS UP 4 STEPS ON HANDS AND KNEES/FEET	0 ☐	1 ☑	2 ☐	3 ☐	46.
47.	4 POINT: CRAWLS BACKWARDS DOWN 4 STEPS ON HANDS AND KNEES/FEET	0 ☑	1 ☐	2 ☐	3 ☐	47.
48.	SIT ON MAT: ATTAINS HIGH KN USING ARMS, MAINTAINS, ARMS FREE, 10 SECONDS	0 ☐	1 ☐	2 ☐	3 ☑	48.
49.	HIGH KN: ATTAINS HALF KN ON R KNEE USING ARMS, MAINTAINS, ARMS FREE, 10 SECONDS	0 ☑	1 ☐	2 ☐	3 ☐	49.
50.	HIGH KN: ATTAINS HALF KN ON L KNEE USING ARMS, MAINTAINS, ARMS FREE, 10 SECONDS	0 ☐	1 ☐	2 ☑	3 ☐	50.
51.	HIGH KN: KN WALKS FORWARD 10 STEPS, ARMS FREE	0 ☑	1 ☐	2 ☐	3 ☐	51.

TOTAL DIMENSION C 25

Item	D: **STANDING**		SCORE			
52.	ON THE FLOOR: PULLS TO STD AT LARGE BENCH	0 ☐	1 ☐	2 ☑	3 ☐	52.
53.	STD: MAINTAINS, ARMS FREE, 3 SECONDS	0 ☐	1 ☐	2 ☑	3 ☐	53.
54.	STD: HOLDING ON TO LARGE BENCH WITH ONE HAND, LIFTS R FOOT, 3 SECONDS	0 ☐	1 ☑	2 ☐	3 ☐	54.
55.	STD: HOLDING ON TO LARGE BENCH WITH ONE HAND, LIFTS L FOOT, 3 SECONDS	0 ☑	1 ☐	2 ☐	3 ☐	55.
56.	STD: MAINTAINS, ARMS FREE, 20 SECONDS	0 ☑	1 ☐	2 ☐	3 ☐	56.
57.	STD: LIFTS L FOOT, ARMS FREE, 10 SECONDS	0 ☑	1 ☐	2 ☐	3 ☐	57.
58.	STD: LIFTS R FOOT, ARMS FREE, 10 SECONDS	0 ☑	1 ☐	2 ☐	3 ☐	58.
59.	SIT ON SMALL BENCH: ATTAINS STD WITHOUT USING ARMS	0 ☑	1 ☐	2 ☐	3 ☐	59.
60.	HIGH KN: ATTAINS STD THROUGH HALF KN ON R KNEE, WITHOUT USING ARMS	0 ☑	1 ☐	2 ☐	3 ☐	60.
61.	HIGH KN: ATTAINS STD THROUGH HALF KN ON L KNEE, WITHOUT USING ARMS	0 ☐	1 ☑	2 ☐	3 ☐	61.
62.	STD: LOWERS TO SIT ON FLOOR WITH CONTROL, ARMS FREE	0 ☑	1 ☐	2 ☐	3 ☐	62.
63.	STD: ATTAINS SQUAT, ARMS FREE	0 ☑	1 ☐	2 ☐	3 ☐	63.
64.	STD: PICKS UP OBJECT FROM FLOOR, ARMS FREE, RETURNS TO STAND	0 ☑	1 ☐	2 ☐	3 ☐	64.

TOTAL DIMENSION D 6

#	Item	0	1	2	3	#
65.	STD, 2 HANDS ON LARGE BENCH: CRUISES 5 STEPS TO R	✓	☐	☐	☐	65.
66.	STD, 2 HANDS ON LARGE BENCH: CRUISES 5 STEPS TO L	✓	☐	☐	☐	66.
67.	STD, 2 HANDS HELD: WALKS FORWARD 10 STEPS	✓	☐	☐	☐	67.
68.	STD, 1 HAND HELD: WALKS FORWARD 10 STEPS	✓	☐	☐	☐	68.
69.	STD: WALKS FORWARD 10 STEPS	✓	☐	☐	☐	69.
70.	STD: WALKS FORWARD 10 STEPS, STOPS, TURNS 180°, RETURNS	✓	☐	☐	☐	70.
71.	STD: WALKS BACKWARD 10 STEPS	✓	☐	☐	☐	71.
72.	STD: WALKS FORWARD 10 STEPS, CARRYING A LARGE OBJECT WITH 2 HANDS	✓	☐	☐	☐	72.
73.	STD: WALKS FORWARD 10 CONSECUTIVE STEPS BETWEEN PARALLEL LINES 8″ APART	✓	☐	☐	☐	73.
74.	STD: WALKS FORWARD 10 CONSECUTIVE STEPS ON A STRAIGHT LINE ¾″ WIDE	✓	☐	☐	☐	74.
75.	STD: STEPS OVER STICK AT KNEE LEVEL, R FOOT LEADING	✓	☐	☐	☐	75.
76.	STD: STEPS OVER STICK AT KNEE LEVEL, L FOOT LEADING	✓	☐	☐	☐	76.
77.	STD: RUNS 15 FEET, STOPS & RETURNS	✓	☐	☐	☐	77.
78.	STD: KICKS BALL WITH R FOOT	✓	☐	☐	☐	78.
79.	STD: KICKS BALL WITH L FOOT	✓	☐	☐	☐	79.
80.	STD: JUMPS 12″ HIGH, BOTH FEET SIMULTANEOUSLY	✓	☐	☐	☐	80.
81.	STD: JUMPS FORWARD 12″, BOTH FEET SIMULTANEOUSLY	✓	☐	☐	☐	81.
82.	STD ON R FOOT: HOPS ON R FOOT 10 TIMES WITHIN A 24″ CIRCLE	✓	☐	☐	☐	82.
83.	STD ON L FOOT: HOPS ON L FOOT 10 TIMES WITHIN A 24″ CIRCLE	✓	☐	☐	☐	83.
84.	STD, HOLDING 1 RAIL: WALKS UP 4 STEPS, HOLDING 1 RAIL, ALTERNATING FEET	✓	☐	☐	☐	84.
85.	STD, HOLDING 1 RAIL: WALKS DOWN 4 STEPS, HOLDING 1 RAIL, ALTERNATING FEET	✓	☐	☐	☐	85.
86.	STD: WALKS UP 4 STEPS, ALTERNATING FEET	✓	☐	☐	☐	86.
87.	STD: WALKS DOWN 4 STEPS, ALTERNATING FEET	✓	☐	☐	☐	87.
88.	STD ON 6″ STEP: JUMPS OFF, BOTH FEET SIMULTANEOUSLY	✓	☐	☐	☐	88.

TOTAL DIMENSION E   [0]

Was this assessment indicative of this child's "regular" performance?   YES [✓] NO ☐

COMMENTS:

Refused   14, 15, 30, 31, 38

GMFM

SUMMARY SCORE

DIMENSION	CALCULATION OF DIMENSION % SCORES	GOAL AREA (Indicated with ✓ check)
A. Lying & Rolling	$\dfrac{\text{Total Dimension A}}{51} = \dfrac{37}{51}$ x 100 = __73__ %	A. ☐
B. Sitting	$\dfrac{\text{Total Dimension B}}{60} = \dfrac{39}{60}$ x 100 = __65__ %	B. ☑
C. Crawling & Kneeling	$\dfrac{\text{Total Dimension C}}{42} = \dfrac{25}{42}$ x 100 = __60__ %	C. ☑
D. Standing	$\dfrac{\text{Total Dimension D}}{39} = \dfrac{6}{39}$ x 100 = __15__ %	D. ☑
E. Walking, Running & Jumping	$\dfrac{\text{Total Dimension E}}{72} = \dfrac{0}{72}$ x 100 = __0__ %	E. ☐

TOTAL SCORE $= \dfrac{\%\ A\ +\ \%\ B\ +\ \%\ C\ +\ \%\ D\ +\ \%\ E}{\text{Total \# of Dimensions}}$

$= \dfrac{73 + 65 + 60 + 15 + 0}{5} = \dfrac{213}{5} = 43\ \%$

GOAL TOTAL SCORE $= \dfrac{\text{Sum of \% scores for each dimension identified as a goal area}}{\text{\# Goal areas}}$

$= \dfrac{65 + 60 + 15}{3} = 47\ \%$

191

TESTING WITH AIDS/ORTHOSES

Indicate below with a check (✓) which aid/orthosis was used and what dimension it was first applied. (There may be more than one).

Aid	Dimension		Orthosis	Dimension
Rollator/pusher............................	☐ _____		Hip Control................................	☐ _____
Walker......................................	☐ _____		Knee Control.............................	☐ _____
H Frame crutches......................	☐ _____		Ankle-foot Control......................	☐ _____
Crutches...................................	☐ _____		Foot Control..............................	☐ _____
Quad Cane...............................	☐ _____		Shoes......................................	☐ _____
Cane..	☐ _____		None.......................................	☑ _____
None..	☑ _____		Other _____	☐ _____
Other _____	☐ _____		(please specify)	
(please specify)				

SUMMARY SCORE USING AIDS/ORTHOSES

DIMENSION	CALCULATION OF DIMENSION % SCORES	GOAL AREA (indicated with ✓ check)
A. Lying & Rolling	$\dfrac{\text{Total Dimension A}}{51} = \dfrac{}{51} \times 100 = \underline{}$ %	A. ☐
B. Sitting	$\dfrac{\text{Total Dimension B}}{60} = \dfrac{}{60} \times 100 = \underline{}$ %	B. ☐
C. Crawling & Kneeling	$\dfrac{\text{Total Dimension C}}{42} = \dfrac{}{42} \times 100 = \underline{}$ %	C. ☐
D. Standing	$\dfrac{\text{Total Dimension D}}{39} = \dfrac{}{39} \times 100 = \underline{}$ %	D. ☐
E. Walking, Running & Jumping	$\dfrac{\text{Total Dimension E}}{72} = \dfrac{}{72} \times 100 = \underline{}$ %	E. ☐

TOTAL SCORE $= \dfrac{\% A + \% B + \% C + \% D + \% E}{\text{Total \# of Dimensions}}$

$$= \frac{ + + + + }{5} = \frac{}{5} = \underline{} \%$$

GOAL TOTAL SCORE $= \dfrac{\text{Sum of \% scores for each dimension identified as a goal area}}{\text{\# Goal areas}}$

$$= \underline{} = \underline{} \%$$

Case Summary Report

Gross Motor Function Measure
GMFM-66

Client ID: 3
Name: Susie Q
Date of Birth: 07 July 1987
Gender: female
Diagnosis: mixed

Assessment Date	Age	GMFM-66 Score	Standard Error	95% Confidence Intervals Lower	Upper	Items Tested	GMFCS	Therapist	Change Score
06 Oct 1989	2y 2m	44.97	1.06	42.89	47.05	64	Level III	Mary Therapist	3.36
03 Apr 1989	1y 8m	41.61	1.14	39.38	43.84	63	Level III	Mary Therapist	N/A

Case Summary Plot:

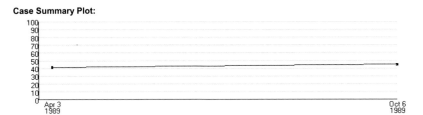

Fig. A3.7. Case summary report after follow-up assessment.

Fig. A3.8. Data from the follow-up assessment as entered into the new score sheet.

GROSS MOTOR FUNCTION MEASURE (GMFM)
SCORE SHEET (GMFM-88 and GMFM-66 scoring)
Version 1.0

Child's Name: _Susie_   ID #: _1234_

Assessment date: _89 / 10 / 06_
       year / month /day

Date of birth: _87 / 07 / 07_
       year / month /day

Chronological age: _2/3_
       years/months

Evaluator's Name: _Mary Therapist_

GMFCS Level [1]

☐ ☐ ☑ ☐ ☐
I   II   III   IV   V

Testing Conditions (eg, room, clothing, time, others present)

Physiotherapy gym   9:30 am
Clothing - diaper, Mom present

The GMFM is a standardized observational instrument designed and validated to measure change in gross motor function over time in children with cerebral palsy. The scoring key is meant to be a general guideline. However, most of the items have specific descriptors for each score. It is imperative that the guidelines contained in the manual be used for scoring each item.

     SCORING KEY   0 = does not initiate
                              1 = initiates
                              2 = partially completes
                              3 = completes
                              NT = Not tested [used for the GMAE scoring*]

It is now important to differentiate a true score of "0" (child does not initiate) from an item which is Not Tested (NT) if you are interested in using the GMFM-66 Ability Estimator Software.

*The GMFM-66 Gross Motor Ability Estimator (GMAE) software is available with the GMFM manual (2002). The advantage of the software is the conversion of the ordinal scale into an interval scale. This will allow for a more accurate estimate of the child's ability and provide a measure that is equally responsive to change across the spectrum of ability levels. Items that are used in the calculation of the GMFM-66 score are shaded and identified with an asterisk (*). The GMFM-66 is only valid for use with children who have cerebral palsy.

Contact for Research Group:
Dianne Russell, *CanChild* Centre for Childhood Disability Research, McMaster University, Institute for Applied Health Sciences, McMaster University, 1400 Main St. W., Rm. 408, Hamilton, L8S 1C7
Tel: North America - 1 905 525-9140 Ext: 27850
Tel: All other countries - 001 905 525-9140 Ext: 27850
E-mail: canchild@mcmaster.ca   Fax: 1 905 522-6095

               Website: www.fhs.mcmaster.ca/canchild

[1] GMFCS level is a rating of severity of motor function. Definitions are found in Appendix I of the GMFM manual (2002).

Check (✓) the appropriate score: if an item is not tested (NT), circle the item number in the right column

Item	A: LYING & ROLLING	SCORE	NT
1.	SUP, HEAD IN MIDLINE: TURNS HEAD WITH EXTREMITIES SYMMETRICAL	0☐ 1☐ 2☐ 3☑	1.
* 2.	SUP: BRINGS HANDS TO MIDLINE, FINGERS ONE WTH THE OTHER	0☐ 1☐ 2☐ 3☑	2.
3.	SUP: LIFTS HEAD 45°	0☐ 1☐ 2☑ 3☐	3.
4.	SUP: FLEXES R HIP AND KNEE THROUGH FULL RANGE	0☐ 1☐ 2☑ 3☐	4.
5.	SUP: FLEXES L HIP AND KNEE THROUGH FULL RANGE	0☐ 1☐ 2☑ 3☐	5.
* 6.	SUP: REACHES OUT WITH R ARM, HAND CROSSES MIDLINE TOWARD TOY	0☐ 1☐ 2☐ 3☑	6.
* 7.	SUP: REACHES OUT WITH L ARM, HAND CROSSES MIDLINE TOWARD TOY	0☐ 1☐ 2☐ 3☑	7.
8.	SUP: ROLLS TO PR OVER R SIDE	0☐ 1☐ 2☐ 3☑	8.
9.	SUP: ROLLS TO PR OVER L SIDE	0☐ 1☐ 2☐ 3☑	9.
* 10.	PR: LIFTS HEAD UPRIGHT	0☐ 1☐ 2☐ 3☑	10.
11.	PR ON FOREARMS: LIFTS HEAD UPRIGHT, ELBOWS EXT., CHEST RAISED	0☐ 1☐ 2☐ 3☑	11.
12.	PR ON FOREARMS: WEIGHT ON R FOREARM, FULLY EXTENDS OPPOSITE ARM FORWARD	0☐ 1☐ 2☑ 3☐	12.
13.	PR ON FOREARMS: WEIGHT ON L FOREARM, FULLY EXTENDS OPPOSITE ARM FORWARD	0☐ 1☐ 2☑ 3☐	13.
14.	PR: ROLLS TO SUP OVER R SIDE	0☐ 1☐ 2☐ 3☐	(14.)
15.	PR: ROLLS TO SUP OVER L SIDE	0☐ 1☐ 2☐ 3☐	(15.)
16.	PR: PIVOTS TO R 90° USING EXTREMITIES	0☐ 1☐ 2☐ 3☑	16.
17.	PR: PIVOTS TO L 90° USING EXTREMITIES	0☑ 1☐ 2☐ 3☐	17.

TOTAL DIMENSION A | 37

Item	B: SITTING	SCORE	NT
* 18.	SUP, HANDS GRASPED BY EXAMINER: PULLS SELF TO SITTING WITH HEAD CONTROL	0☐ 1☐ 2☐ 3☑	18.
19.	SUP: ROLLS TO R SIDE, ATTAINS SITTING	0☑ 1☐ 2☐ 3☐	19.
20.	SUP: ROLLS TO L SIDE, ATTAINS SITTING	0☑ 1☐ 2☐ 3☐	20.
* 21.	SIT ON MAT, SUPPORTED AT THORAX BY THERAPIST: LIFTS HEAD UPRIGHT, MAINTAINS 3 SECONDS	0☐ 1☐ 2☐ 3☑	21.
* 22.	SIT ON MAT, SUPPORTED AT THORAX BY THERAPIST: LIFTS HEAD MIDLINE, MAINTAINS 10 SECONDS	0☐ 1☐ 2☑ 3☐	22.
* 23.	SIT ON MAT, ARM(S) PROPPING: MAINTAINS, 5 SECONDS	0☐ 1☐ 2☐ 3☑	23.
* 24.	SIT ON MAT: MAINTAIN, ARMS FREE, 3 SECONDS	0☐ 1☐ 2☐ 3☑	24.
* 25.	SIT ON MAT WITH SMALL TOY IN FRONT: LEANS FORWARD, TOUCHES TOY, RE-ERECTS WITHOUT ARM PROPPING	0☐ 1☐ 2☑ 3☐	25.
* 26.	SIT ON MAT: TOUCHES TOY PLACED 45° BEHIND CHILD'S R SIDE, RETURNS TO START	0☐ 1☐ 2☐ 3☑	26.
* 27.	SIT ON MAT: TOUCHES TOY PLACED 45° BEHIND CHILD'S L SIDE, RETURNS TO START	0☐ 1☑ 2☐ 3☐	27.
28.	R SIDE SIT: MAINTAINS, ARMS FREE, 5 SECONDS	0☐ 1☐ 2☐ 3☑	28.
29.	L SIDE SIT: MAINTAINS, ARMS FREE, 5 SECONDS	0☐ 1☐ 2☐ 3☑	29.
* 30.	SIT ON MAT: LOWERS TO PR WITH CONTROL	0☐ 1☐ 2☐ 3☐	(30.)
* 31.	SIT ON MAT WITH FEET IN FRONT: ATTAINS 4 POINT OVER R SIDE	0☐ 1☐ 2☐ 3☐	(31.)
* 32.	SIT ON MAT WITH FEET IN FRONT: ATTAINS 4 POINT OVER L SIDE	0☐ 1☐ 2☐ 3☑	32.
33.	SIT ON MAT: PIVOTS 90°, WITHOUT ARMS ASSISTING	0☐ 1☐ 2☑ 3☐	33.
34.	SIT ON BENCH: MAINTAINS, ARMS AND FEET FREE, 10 SECONDS	0☐ 1☐ 2☑ 3☐	34.
* 35.	STD: ATTAINS SIT ON SMALL BENCH	0☐ 1☐ 2☑ 3☐	35.
* 36.	ON THE FLOOR: ATTAINS SIT ON SMALL BENCH	0☐ 1☐ 2☑ 3☐	36.
* 37.	ON THE FLOOR: ATTAINS SIT ON LARGE BENCH	0☐ 1☐ 2☑ 3☐	37.

TOTAL DIMENSION B | 39

GMFM SCORE SHEET

Item	C: CRAWLING & KNEELING		SCORE				NT
38.	PR: CREEPS FORWARD 1.8m (6')	0 ☐	1 ☐	2 ☐	3 ☐		(38)
* 39.	4 POINT: MAINTAINS, WEIGHT ON HANDS AND KNEES, 10 SECONDS	0 ☐	1 ☐	2 ☐	3 ☑		39.
* 40.	4 POINT: ATTAINS SIT ARMS FREE	0 ☐	1 ☐	2 ☑	3 ☐		40.
* 41.	PR: ATTAINS 4 POINT, WEIGHT ON HANDS AND KNEES	0 ☐	1 ☐	2 ☐	3 ☑		41.
* 42.	4 POINT: REACHES FORWARD WITH R ARM, HAND ABOVE SHOULDER LEVEL	0 ☐	1 ☐	2 ☐	3 ☑		42.
* 43.	4 POINT: REACHES FORWARD WITH L ARM, HAND ABOVE SHOULDER LEVEL	0 ☐	1 ☐	2 ☐	3 ☑		43.
* 44.	4 POINT: CRAWLS OR HITCHES FORWARD 1.8m (6')	0 ☐	1 ☐	2 ☐	3 ☑		44.
* 45.	4 POINT: CRAWLS RECIPROCALLY FORWARD 1.8m (6')	0 ☐	1 ☐	2 ☑	3 ☐		45.
* 46.	4 POINT: CRAWLS UP 4 STEPS ON HANDS AND KNEES/FEET	0 ☐	1 ☑	2 ☐	3 ☐		46.
47.	4 POINT: CRAWLS BACKWARDS DOWN 4 STEPS ON HANDS AND KNEES/FEET	0 ☑	1 ☐	2 ☐	3 ☐		47.
* 48.	SIT ON MAT: ATTAINS HIGH KN USING ARMS, MAINTAINS, ARMS FREE, 10 SECONDS	0 ☐	1 ☐	2 ☐	3 ☑		48.
49.	HIGH KN: ATTAINS HALF KN ON R KNEE USING ARMS, MAINTAINS, ARMS FREE, 10 SECONDS	0 ☑	1 ☐	2 ☐	3 ☐		49.
50.	HIGH KN: ATTAINS HALF KN ON L KNEE USING ARMS, MAINTAINS, ARMS FREE, 10 SECONDS	0 ☐	1 ☐	2 ☑	3 ☐		50.
* 51.	HIGH KN: KN WALKS FORWARD 10 STEPS, ARMS FREE	0 ☑	1 ☐	2 ☐	3 ☐		51.

TOTAL DIMENSION C 25

Item	D: STANDING		SCORE				NT
* 52.	ON THE FLOOR: PULLS TO STD AT LARGE BENCH	0 ☐	1 ☐	2 ☑	3 ☐		52.
* 53.	STD: MAINTAINS, ARMS FREE, 3 SECONDS	0 ☐	1 ☐	2 ☑	3 ☐		53.
* 54.	STD: HOLDING ON TO LARGE BENCH WITH ONE HAND, LIFTS R FOOT, 3 SECONDS	0 ☐	1 ☑	2 ☐	3 ☐		54.
* 55.	STD: HOLDING ON TO LARGE BENCH WITH ONE HAND, LIFTS R FOOT, 3 SECONDS	0 ☑	1 ☐	2 ☐	3 ☐		55.
* 56.	STD: MAINTAINS, ARMS FREE, 20 SECONDS	0 ☑	1 ☐	2 ☐	3 ☐		56.
* 57.	STD: LIFTS L FOOT, ARMS FREE, 10 SECONDS	0 ☑	1 ☐	2 ☐	3 ☐		57.
* 58.	STD: LIFTS R FOOT, ARMS FREE, 10 SECONDS	0 ☑	1 ☐	2 ☐	3 ☐		58.
* 59.	SIT ON SMALL BENCH: ATTAINS STD WITHOUT USING ARMS	0 ☑	1 ☐	2 ☐	3 ☐		59.
* 60.	HIGH KN: ATTAINS STD THROUGH HALF KN ON R KNEE, WITHOUT USING ARMS	0 ☐	1 ☑	2 ☐	3 ☐		60.
* 61.	HIGH KN: ATTAINS STD THROUGH HALF KN ON L KNEE, WITHOUT USING ARMS	0 ☑	1 ☐	2 ☐	3 ☐		61.
* 62.	STD: LOWERS TO SIT ON FLOOR WITH CONTROL, ARMS FREE	0 ☑	1 ☐	2 ☐	3 ☐		62.
* 63.	STD: ATTAINS SQUAT, ARMS FREE	0 ☑	1 ☐	2 ☐	3 ☐		63.
* 64.	STD: PICKS UP OBJECT FROM FLOOR, ARMS FREE, RETURNS TO STAND	0 ☑	1 ☐	2 ☐	3 ☐		64.

TOTAL DIMENSION D 6

Item	E: WALKING, RUNNING & JUMPING	SCORE	NT
65.	STD, 2 HANDS ON LARGE BENCH: CRUISES 5 STEPS TO R.............................	0 ☑ 1 ☐ 2 ☐ 3 ☐	65.
66.	STD, 2 HANDS ON LARGE BENCH: CRUISES 5 STEPS TO L	0 ☑ 1 ☐ 2 ☐ 3 ☐	66.
67.	STD, 2 HANDS HELD: WALKS FORWARD 10 STEPS....................................	0 ☑ 1 ☐ 2 ☐ 3 ☐	67.
68.	STD, 1 HAND HELD: WALKS FORWARD 10 STEPS	0 ☑ 1 ☐ 2 ☐ 3 ☐	68.
69.	STD: WALKS FORWARD 10 STEPS...	0 ☑ 1 ☐ 2 ☐ 3 ☐	69.
70.	STD: WALKS FORWARD 10 STEPS, STOPS, TURNS 180°, RETURNS	0 ☐ 1 ☐ 2 ☐ 3 ☐	(70.)
71.	STD: WALKS BACKWARD 10 STEPS	0 ☐ 1 ☐ 2 ☐ 3 ☐	(71.)
72.	STD: WALKS FORWARD 10 STEPS, CARRYING A LARGE OBJECT WITH 2 HANDS	0 ☐ 1 ☐ 2 ☐ 3 ☐	(72.)
73.	STD: WALKS FORWARD 10 CONSECUTIVE STEPS BETWEEN PARALLEL LINES 20cm (8") APART	0 ☐ 1 ☐ 2 ☐ 3 ☐	(73.)
74.	STD: WALKS FORWARD 10 CONSECUTIVE STEPS ON A STRAIGHT LINE 2cm (3/4") WIDE........	0 ☐ 1 ☐ 2 ☐ 3 ☐	(74.)
75.	STD: STEPS OVER STICK AT KNEE LEVEL, R FOOT LEADING............................	0 ☐ 1 ☐ 2 ☐ 3 ☐	(75.)
76.	STD: STEPS OVER STICK AT KNEE LEVEL, L FOOT LEADING	0 ☐ 1 ☐ 2 ☐ 3 ☐	(76.)
77.	STD: RUNS 4.5m (15'), STOPS & RETURNS	0 ☐ 1 ☐ 2 ☐ 3 ☐	(77.)
78.	STD: KICKS BALL WITH R FOOT	0 ☐ 1 ☐ 2 ☐ 3 ☐	(78.)
79.	STD: KICKS BALL WITH L FOOT	0 ☐ 1 ☐ 2 ☐ 3 ☐	(79.)
80.	STD: JUMPS 30cm (12") HIGH, BOTH FEET SIMULTANEOUSLY............................	0 ☐ 1 ☐ 2 ☐ 3 ☐	(80.)
81.	STD: JUMPS FORWARD 30 cm (12"), BOTH FEET SIMULTANEOUSLY	0 ☐ 1 ☐ 2 ☐ 3 ☐	(81.)
82.	STD ON R FOOT: HOPS ON R FOOT 10 TIMES WITHIN A 60cm (24") CIRCLE	0 ☐ 1 ☐ 2 ☐ 3 ☐	(82.)
83.	STD ON L FOOT: HOPS ON L FOOT 10 TIMES WITHIN A 60cm (24") CIRCLE	0 ☐ 1 ☐ 2 ☐ 3 ☐	(83.)
84.	STD, HOLDING 1 RAIL: WALKS UP 4 STEPS, HOLDING 1 RAIL, ALTERNATING FEET.........	0 ☐ 1 ☐ 2 ☐ 3 ☐	(84.)
85.	STD, HOLDING 1 RAIL: WALKS DOWN 4 STEPS, HOLDING 1 RAIL, ALTERNATING FEET	0 ☐ 1 ☐ 2 ☐ 3 ☐	(85.)
86.	STD: WALKS UP 4 STEPS, ALTERNATING FEET.....................................	0 ☐ 1 ☐ 2 ☐ 3 ☐	(86.)
87.	STD: WALKS DOWN 4 STEPS, ALTERNATING FEET....................................	0 ☐ 1 ☐ 2 ☐ 3 ☐	(87.)
88.	STD ON 15cm (6") STEP: JUMPS OFF, BOTH FEET SIMULTANEOUSLY	0 ☐ 1 ☐ 2 ☐ 3 ☐	(88.)

TOTAL DIMENSION E [   ]

Was this assessment indicative of this child's "regular" performance?   YES ☑ NO ☐

COMMENTS:

_____

_____

_____

_____

_____

_____

_____

_____

GMFM SCORE SHEET

GMFM RAW SUMMARY SCORE

DIMENSION	CALCULATION OF DIMENSION % SCORES	GOAL AREA (indicated with ✓ check)

A. Lying & Rolling $\dfrac{\text{Total Dimension A}}{51} = \dfrac{37}{51} \times 100 = \underline{73}$ %   A. ☐

B. Sitting $\dfrac{\text{Total Dimension B}}{60} = \dfrac{39}{60} \times 100 = \underline{65}$ %   B. ☑

C. Crawling & Kneeling $\dfrac{\text{Total Dimension C}}{42} = \dfrac{25}{42} \times 100 = \underline{60}$ %   C. ☑

D. Standing $\dfrac{\text{Total Dimension D}}{39} = \dfrac{6}{39} \times 100 = \underline{15}$ %   D. ☑

E. Walking, Running & Jumping $\dfrac{\text{Total Dimension E}}{72} = \dfrac{0}{72} \times 100 = \underline{0}$ %   E. ☐

TOTAL SCORE = $\dfrac{\%A + \%B + \%C + \%D + \%E}{\text{Total \# of Dimensions}}$

$$= \frac{73 + 65 + 60 + 15 + 0}{5} = \frac{213}{5} = \underline{43}\ \%$$

GOAL TOTAL SCORE = $\dfrac{\text{Sum of \% scores for each dimension identified as a goal area}}{\text{\# of Goal areas}}$

$$= \frac{65 + 60 + 15}{3} = \underline{47}\ \%$$

GMFM-66 Gross Motor Ability Estimator Score [1]

GMFM-66 Score = $\underline{44.97}$ $\underline{42.89}$ to $\underline{47.05}$
95% Confidence Intervals

previous GMFM-66 Score = $\underline{41.61}$ $\underline{39.38}$ to $\underline{43.84}$
95% Confidence Intervals

change in GMFM-66 = $\underline{3.36}$

[1] from the Gross Motor Ability Estimator (GMAE) Software

TESTING WITH AIDS/ORTHOSES

Indicate below with a check (✓) which aid/orthosis was used and what dimension it was first applied. (There may be more than one).

AID	DIMENSION	ORTHOSIS	DIMENSION
Rollator/Pusher..............................	☐ ____	Hip Control..	☐ ____
Walker...	☐ ____	Knee Control.....................................	☐ ____
H Frame Crutches..........................	☐ ____	Ankle-Foot Control............................	☐ ____
Crutches	☐ ____	Foot Control	☐ ____
Quad Cane	☐ ____	Shoes...	☐ ____
Cane	☐ ____	None	☑ ____
None	☑ ____	Other	☐ ____
Other	☐ ____	(please specify)	

(please specify)

RAW SUMMARY SCORE USING AIDS/ORTHOSES

DIMENSION	CALCULATION OF DIMENSION % SCORES	GOAL AREA (indicated with ✓ check)

F. Lying & Rolling $\dfrac{\text{Total Dimension A}}{51}$ = $\dfrac{}{51}$ × 100 = _____ %   A. ☐

G. Sitting $\dfrac{\text{Total Dimension B}}{60}$ = $\dfrac{}{60}$ × 100 = _____ %   B. ☐

H. Crawling & Kneeling $\dfrac{\text{Total Dimension C}}{42}$ = $\dfrac{}{42}$ × 100 = _____ %   C. ☐

I. Standing $\dfrac{\text{Total Dimension D}}{39}$ = $\dfrac{}{39}$ × 100 = _____ %   D. ☐

J. Walking, Running & Jumping $\dfrac{\text{Total Dimension E}}{72}$ = $\dfrac{}{72}$ × 100 = _____ %   E. ☐

TOTAL SCORE = $\dfrac{\text{\%A + \%B + \%C + \%D + \%E}}{\text{Total \# of Dimensions}}$

= $\dfrac{\_\_ + \_\_ + \_\_ + \_\_ + \_\_}{5}$ = $\dfrac{}{5}$ = _____ %

GOAL TOTAL SCORE = $\dfrac{\text{Sum of \% scores for each dimension identified as a goal area}}{\text{\# of Goal areas}}$

= $\dfrac{}{}$ = _____ %

GMFM-66 Gross Motor Ability Estimator Score [1]

GMFM-66 Score = _____   _____ to _____
                                        95% Confidence Intervals

previous GMFM-66 Score = _____   _____ to _____
                                        95% Confidence Intervals

change in GMFM-66 = _____

[1] from the Gross Motor Ability Estimator (GMAE) Software

APPENDIX 4
GMFM-66 AND GMFM-88 CROSS-SECTIONAL AND CHANGE SCORES

This appendix presents, in tabular and graphical form, the mean and median scores on the GMFM-66 and GMFM-88 of a sample of children with cerebral palsy (CP), categorized by age group and severity of CP as judged using the Gross Motor Function Classification System (GMFCS), and the mean and median change scores at follow-up testing six months and 12 months after the initial assessments.

TABLE A4.1
Mean and median GMFM-66 scores for children with CP by age category and GMFCS severity level*

Age (years)	GMFCS level					Total
	Level I	Level II	Level III	Level IV	Level V	
<2	55.6	43.8	39.3	27.8	21.9	41.0
	(6.5)	—	(7.3)	(5.3)	(2.4)	(14.3)
	57.4	43.8	42.9	27.6	20.5	43.4
	8	1	5	4	3	21
2–4	65.6	51.3	47.5	34.8	20.0	44.8
	(9.9)	(6.8)	(4.2)	(6.9)	(7.5)	(17.4)
	66.3	52.0	47.7	35.7	20.5	46.9
	25	26	19	19	22	111
4–6	73.5	60.8	51.4	41.6	24.3	51.7
	(9.5)	(7.6)	(7.7)	(6.3)	(7.2)	(20.1)
	73.6	61.2	51.6	43.1	23.4	50.2
	48	10	23	34	29	144
>6	84.1	68.0	51.8	39.3	22.0	54.0
	(9.0)	(7.8)	(6.3)	(7.1)	(9.7)	(24.2)
	84.1	67.2	52.5	39.2	22.3	52.0
	103	44	76	79	74	376
Total	77.6	61.5	50.5	38.9	22.2	51.5
	(12.3)	(10.7)	(6.8)	(7.3)	(8.8)	(22.3)
	79.1	62.4	50.9	39.2	22.0	49.9
	184	81	123	136	128	652

*Each block of four numbers represents, from the top down, the mean score, the standard deviation from the mean, the median score, and the number of children assessed in that category.

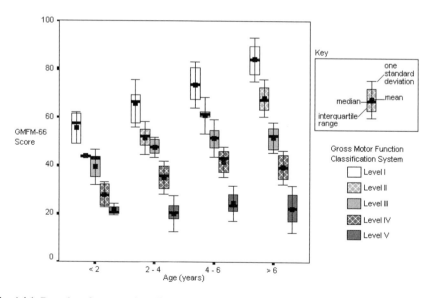

Fig. A4.1. Box plot of mean and median GMFM-66 scores for children with CP by age category and GMFCS severity level.

Mean and median GMFM-88 scores for children with CP by age category and GMFCS severity level*

Age (years)	GMFCS level					Total
	Level I	Level II	Level III	Level IV	Level V	
<2	69.9	50.3	37.7	21.1	8.9	43.3
	(11.6)	—	(14.2)	(5.2)	(0.4)	(25.7)
	72.8	50.3	42.6	22.4	8.7	45.3
	8	1	5	4	3	21
2–4	81.2	61.2	54.3	28.4	9.9	48.8
	(13.5)	(14.9)	(10.5)	(9.2)	(5.8)	(28.0)
	86.0	64.7	55.8	27.9	9.4	54.1
	25	26	19	19	22	111
4–6	90.8	75.8	62.0	40.4	15.3	58.0
	(8.6)	(16.3)	(15.3)	(12.9)	(7.7)	(30.9)
	93.1	80.1	64.6	43.1	13.3	61.1
	48	10	23	34	29	144
>6	96.8	85.9	62.3	36.0	13.3	59.4
	(3.3)	(9.5)	(13.2)	(14.0)	(9.4)	(33.3)
	97.8	87.5	65.1	32.9	12.7	63.7
	103	44	76	79	74	376
Total	92.0	76.3	60.0	35.6	13.1	56.7
	(10.2)	(16.8)	(14.2)	(13.6)	(8.5)	(32.0)
	96.2	81.7	61.6	32.4	11.5	59.2
	184	81	123	136	128	652

*Each block of four numbers represents, from the top down, the mean score, the standard deviation from the mean score, the median score, and the number of children assessed in that category.

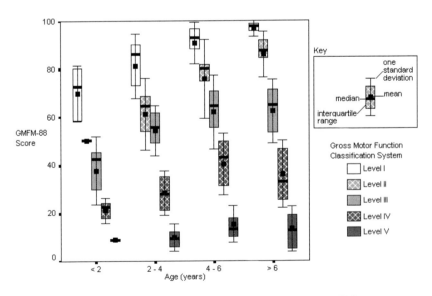

Fig. A4.2. Box plot of mean and median GMFM-88 scores for children with CP by age category and GMFCS severity level

Table of mean and median GMFM-66 and GMFM-88 change scores over six months by age category and GMFCS severity level*

Age (years)	GMFCS level					Total
	Level I	Level II	Level III	Level IV	Level V	
A. GMFM-66 change scores						
<2	5.50	4.12	6.00	−1.06	2.24	4.34
	(2.73)	—	(3.36)	—	(4.83)	(3.57)
	5.68	4.12	7.36	−1.06	0.71	4.36
	6	1	3	1	3	14
2–4	3.22	3.03	2.43	2.63	2.92	2.86
	(2.95)	(3.39)	(2.75)	(3.07)	(4.22)	(3.23)
	2.50	2.00	2.01	2.65	2.06	2.24
	16	16	14	15	14	75
4–6	2.77	0.96	0.02	0.71	1.50	1.42
	(5.01)	(2.90)	(2.99)	(2.49)	(2.28)	(3.66)
	1.82	1.00	0.00	0.94	1.53	1.12
	35	10	17	30	18	110
>6	—	—	0.53	—	3.53	2.03
	—	—	—	—	—	(2.12)
	—	—	0.53	—	3.53	2.03
	—	—	1	—	1	2
Total	3.18	2.30	1.51	1.31	2.17	2.17
	(4.35)	(3.27)	(3.32)	(2.81)	(3.32)	(3.58)
	2.47	1.36	1.01	1.24	1.86	1.68
	57	27	35	46	36	201
B. GMFM-88 change scores						
<2	7.50	7.19	11.03	−5.12	5.03	6.80
	(4.24)	—	(8.52)	—	(5.93)	(6.29)
	6.50	7.19	11.51	−5.12	3.92	6.32
	6	1	3	1	3	14
2–4	2.51	5.31	4.93	5.69	2.08	4.12
	(3.49)	(6.06)	(5.96)	(6.09)	(3.37)	(5.24)
	2.82	4.58	4.10	4.01	0.82	3.24
	16	16	14	15	14	75
4–6	1.24	1.87	0.45	1.29	11.86	2.96
	(3.55)	(2.37)	(4.54)	(3.55)	(42.14)	(17.58)
	1.11	1.36	1.68	1.64	2.19	1.39
	35	10	17	30	18	110
>6	—	—	−0.56	—	3.29	1.37
	—	—	—	—	—	(2.73)
	—	—	−0.56	—	3.29	1.37
	—	—	1	—	1	2
Total	2.27	4.11	3.12	2.62	7.25	3.65
	(4.02)	(5.13)	(6.19)	(5.06)	(29.86)	(13.45)
	1.39	1.85	2.69	2.03	1.69	1.81
	57	27	35	46	36	201

*Each block of four numbers represents, from the top down, the mean score, the standard deviation from the mean, the median score, and the number of children assessed in that category.

Table of mean and median GMFM-66 and GMFM-88 change scores over 12 months by age category and GMFCS severity level*

Age (years)	GMFCS level					Total
	Level I	Level II	Level III	Level IV	Level V	
A. GMFM-66 change scores						
<2	11.57	7.06	8.12	—	—	9.94
	(3.16)	—	(3.49)	—	—	(3.36)
	12.78	7.06	8.12	—	—	10.59
	4	1	2	—	—	7
2–4	4.54	5.46	1.86	4.00	0.97	3.33
	(3.61)	(5.11)	(3.05)	(3.86)	(5.49)	(4.44)
	4.65	4.51	2.17	3.44	1.41	3.06
	13	12	15	10	11	61
4–6	4.58	2.23	2.50	1.48	0.74	2.70
	(5.93)	(6.48)	(2.47)	(2.46)	(5.39)	(5.03)
	4.06	1.88	1.50	0.59	0.00	1.88
	26	9	10	17	11	73
>6	2.49	2.04	0.90	0.43	0.85	1.29
	(4.30)	(5.08)	(3.20)	(2.64)	(3.91)	(3.86)
	1.06	2.00	0.79	0.24	0.71	0.82
	53	33	50	55	49	240
Total	3.71	2.91	1.48	1.08	0.85	2.05
	(5.01)	(5.40)	(3.28)	(2.98)	(4.36)	(4.39)
	3.27	2.06	1.17	0.74	0.71	1.30
	96	55	77	82	71	381
B. GMFM-88 change scores						
<2	14.47	14.97	12.57	—	—	14.00
	(8.40)	—	(6.00)	—	—	(6.50)
	13.29	14.97	12.57	—	—	14.97
	4	1	2	—	—	7
2–4	5.49	8.74	3.67	8.06	2.22	5.52
	(4.61)	(8.03)	(8.48)	(5.44)	(5.45)	(6.94)
	4.94	4.90	3.71	8.10	1.57	4.76
	13	12	15	10	11	61
4–6	3.09	4.62	4.47	2.66	16.48	5.38
	(4.93)	(5.69)	(5.24)	(4.39)	(54.49)	(21.33)
	1.43	4.75	3.32	1.39	1.66	1.66
	26	9	10	17	11	73
>6	0.49	1.55	1.89	1.40	0.19	1.07
	(1.30)	(7.06)	(4.85)	(5.55)	(2.86)	(4.57)
	0.28	1.40	2.02	1.20	0.32	0.69
	53	33	50	55	49	240
Total	2.45	3.87	2.85	2.47	3.03	2.85
	(4.67)	(7.64)	(5.98)	(5.68)	(21.64)	(10.69)
	0.78	3.25	2.23	1.34	0.55	1.30
	96	55	77	82	71	381

*Each block of four numbers represents, from the top down, the mean score, the standard deviation from the mean, the median score, and the number of children assessed in that category.

APPENDIX 5
STANDARD ERROR OF MEASUREMENT

The standard error provided within the item response theory framework is the standard error of the score and is only a small part of the measurement error. The total error in the GMFM-66 score may be described as follows:

$$Total\ error = Error_{assessment} + Error_{estimation} + Error_{calibration}$$

$Error_{assessment}$: The error that arises during the assessment of the child. This error could be caused by the therapist failing to notice a child's movements, incorrectly recording a score on the score sheet or incorrectly entering a score into the computer, and also by the scoring variation among therapists.

$Error_{estimation}$: The error in estimating the GMFM-66 score from the responses to the items tested. This error has not been quantified.

$Error_{calibration}$: The asymptotic error of the estimation process. This is a measure of how evenly the subjects are distributed around the score. Once the original Rasch analysis is complete this error is fixed and is specific to the child's *score* and *not* to the child or to the child's response pattern.

The GMAE provides only the $Error_{calibration}$ part of the total error and this is specified throughout the program as the standard error.

APPENDIX 6
METHODS OF DISPLAYING ITEM DIFFICULTY

Schematic of GMFM-66 item difficulty

A number of methods are available for assessing item difficulty within the framework of item response theory, including (1) step measures, (2) Thurstone thresholds, and (3) expected scores. The discussion of these different methods is complex but important in terms of understanding the concept of probability models, and to gain a good understanding of what is being presented in the item maps. The goal of this discussion is to provide the reader with a brief background to the three common expressions of item difficulty and to clarify where these have been used in the presentation of the GMFM-66.

A discussion of these different methods is facilitated by an examination of item probability curves. Figure A6.1 illustrates the probability curves for each of the four scores on a hypothetical item. These curves show the probability (on the vertical axis) of achieving a score as a function of ability (shown on the horizontal axis, and equivalent to the GMFM-66 score). The far left curve represents the probability of scoring a 0 on the item, P_0. From this curve you can see that a child is most likely to score a 0 when their overall ability is very low. The next leftmost curve, P_1, represents the likelihood of scoring a 1. This is initially very low (when the child's overall ability is low), but as the child's ability increases a score of 1 becomes more likely and reaches a maximum at a GMFM ability score of approximately 45. As the child becomes more able the likelihood increases that s/he will score 2 or 3, and the likelihood of scoring a 1 decreases. The next curve, P_2, represents the likelihood of scoring a 2 and behaves in much the same way as P_1, with the chance of success being initially very low and increasing to a maximum at 54 before decreasing as a score of 3 becomes more likely. Finally, the right-most curve, P_3, represents the likelihood of scoring a 3, which increases as the overall ability of a child increases.

Item step measures

The Rasch analysis computer program (Bigsteps) provides information on the difficulty of each "step" or response option within an item. In the GMFM-66 we have decided *not* to present these "step measures" or difficulties; however, they are a useful concept and perhaps the most easily understood method from a statistical point of view. Step measures indicate the ability level at which a child becomes equally likely to score in adjacent categories for an item. For instance, the item step measure for a score of 1 indicates the ability at which a score of 1 becomes as likely as a score of 0.

On the figure of probability curves (Fig. A6.1) this is where the solid curves intersect each other. If a child has an ability score of 42 on our hypothetical item, then they are equally as likely to score a 0 as a 1. If they have an ability score of 49, then they are equally likely to score a 1 as a 2, and if they score 58 they would have the same probability of scoring a 2 as a 3.

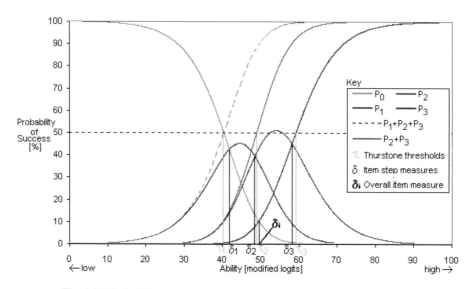

Fig. A6.1. Probability curves for a hypothetical item with four response options.

Thurstone thresholds

The Thurstone thresholds are perhaps the most clinically intuitive method of expressing item difficulty for measures with ordered categories like the GMFM. Thurstone thresholds define the ability at which a child is "likely" (probability $\geq 50\%$) to score in *at least* the category of interest. For instance, a Thurstone threshold for a score of 2 would indicate the ability level at which you would expect a child to score at least a 2 (so either a 2 *or* a 3). The Thurstone thresholds are determined by summing the probability of achieving all scores at and above the score of interest and finding the intersection of this curve and the line of 50% probability ($p=0.5$). Thus, the Thurstone threshold for a score of 2 is defined as the ability where the curve expressing the likelihood of scoring a 2 *or* a 3 (the solid grey curve P_2+P_3 in Fig. A6.1) rises above 50%. On Figure A6.1 the Thurstone threshold for a score of 2 is approximately 49. It is at this ability where the child is likely to be able to score at least a 2 on this item. The broken grey curve in Figure A6.1, $P_1+P_2+P_3$, illustrates the likelihood of scoring a 1 *or* a 2 *or* a 3 and is used to determine the Thurstone threshold for a score of 1. In this example a Thurstone threshold for a score of 1 is 44.5. Finally, when a child's ability is approximately 58 the curve P3 rises above 50% and at this ability a child becomes likely to be able to score a 3 on the item.

The Thurstone thresholds are by convention always set to the point where the probability of success exceeds 50%. This is a useful threshold because, technically, where the probability exceeds 50% is where success becomes "likely". It is possible to use thresholds that use a stricter definition of "likely". In Table 4.4 we have provided both the Thurstone thresholds and the higher threshold of *90% likelihood* to convey the difficulty of completing the GMFM-66 items (completion defined as scoring 3). While technically a child becomes

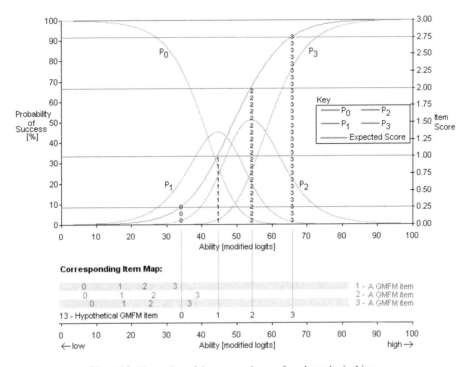

Fig. A6.2. Illustration of the expected score for a hypothetical item.

likely to complete an item with an ability greater than the Thurstone threshold, a child is certainly *more likely* to be able to complete the item at the 90% likelihood threshold.

Expected scores

The difficulties of items may also be expressed with the use of expected scores. The expected scores are the least intuitive method of reporting item difficulty but because they have been used to report item difficulty for at least two other pediatric outcome measures, the Pediatric Evaluation of Disability Inventory (Haley *et al*. 1992) and the School Function Assessment (Coster *et al*. 1998), we felt it was important to be consistent. We have therefore used expected scores for the item maps of the GMFM-66 produced from the GMAE program.

Figure A6.2 provides an example of how an item is displayed on the GMFM-66 item maps using expected scores. This example uses a hypothetical item, with the same characteristics of the item used in Figure A6.1 so that direct comparisons between graphs may be made. This item was designed to provide a clear explanation of the Rasch model and measures of item difficulty and is not a GMFM-66 item.

Figure A6.2 illustrates the expected scores for each of the four possible scores for a hypothetical item. The columns of numbers running vertically down the graph indicate where on an item map the scores for this item would be placed. The probability curves for each of the four scores have been included for comparison with Figure A6.1. The red line indicates the expected score and ranges continuously from 0 to 3. This curve must be read from the right-hand vertical axis.

The concept of "expected" values is common in mathematics and physics but warrants some explanation in this context. The expected score is defined as the sum for all scores of the likelihood of the score multiplied by the value of the score. For the four-point rating scale of the GMFM this means that the expected score is as follows:

$$Expected\ Score = 0 \cdot P_0 + 1 \cdot P_1 + 2 \cdot P_2 + 3 \cdot P_3$$

This makes more sense than a first glance would suggest, but first a little more discussion of expected scores is required.

In general, the "expected value" of any measure is the population mean of that measure. Thus, if the average height of all people (of all ages) in Canada is 1.5 m then we say that the "expected" height of a Canadian is 1.5 m. Obviously in the case of height there is a large population variance and so perhaps this expected score is not very useful. If, however, we could refine our population and instead of looking at all Canadians we just looked at those Canadians aged between, say, 4 and 6 months, then the average height of the population becomes a reasonable estimate of what we would expect for any single person. When we talk about expected scores on the GMFM-66 we talk about the expected score of a child conditional on their ability. Thus, when we say that the expected score of a child with a GMFM-66 score of 30 is 2 on an item what it implies is that if *all children* with cerebral palsy *who score 30* on the GMFM-66 were tested on *that* item, their *average* score would be 2.

Now let us go back to the formula for the expected score:

$$Expected\ Score = 0 \cdot P_0 + 1 \cdot P_1 + 2 \cdot P_2 + 3 \cdot P_3$$

At first glance this doesn't look very much like an average. However, when we consider exactly what it is these probabilities represent the picture becomes a little clearer. Let us assume that we have the entire population available to study. The proportion of all children who score a 0 will be the number of children who score a 0, divided by the total number in the population. If we were to randomly draw a child from this population the probability of the child having a score of 0 would be the proportion of the population who scored 0. Applying this logic to the other probabilities we have:

$$Expected\ Score = 0 \cdot \frac{\#\ of\ children\ scoring\ 0}{Total\ number\ of\ children} + 1 \cdot \frac{\#\ of\ children\ scoring\ 1}{Total\ number\ of\ children}$$

$$+ 2 \cdot \frac{\#\ of\ children\ scoring\ 2}{Total\ number\ of\ children} + 3 \cdot \frac{\#\ of\ children\ scoring\ 3}{Total\ number\ of\ children}$$

Recognizing that the numerators are the total values for each score we get:

$$Expected\ Score = \frac{Sum\ of\ all\ scores}{Total\ number\ of\ children}$$

This, finally, is something we can recognize as the mean score. The expected score is the mean score of the *population*. In our case the population is *all* children with cerebral palsy, and instead of using the population proportions we have estimated these probabilities based on the item step difficulties supplied by the Rasch model. In chapter 4 we presented evidence of the high reliability of these item step difficulties. The high reliability of these item difficulties allows us to be confident that our expected scores accurately estimate the population mean.

With a better understanding of expected scores the item maps can be better understood. The item maps show the ability at which a given score is "expected". For scores of 1 and 2 this is relatively straight-forward. A "1" on the item map indicates the ability at which a score of 1 is expected. Locating a score of 1 on the right-hand vertical axis we follow this across until we encounter the red, expected score curve; we then look down to the horizontal axis and read the ability level. On Figure A6.2 we can see that the expected score of 1 occurs at an ability of about 45. The line of 1's running down the graph indicates that this is where the 1 would be shown on the item map for this item. Using the same process we look across from the "2" on the right-hand vertical axis and see that this intersects the expect score curve at an ability of about 54. Again, there is a line of 2's running down the graph, indicating the location of the 2 on the item map. Now, look at the line of 3's running down the graph. Find the intersection of this line of 3's with the expected score curve and then draw a line over to the right-hand axis. The location of the 3's does not correspond to an expected score of 3, but rather to an expected score of 2.75. An expected score of 3 will only ever occur when the child's ability is 100. This is because only a population of children with perfect scores could have a mean score of 3 on every item. For all other groups the population mean score, and therefore the expected score, will be less than 3. Because placing all the 3's at a score of 100 on the item map would not provide any useful information, it is convention to display the extreme scores 0.25 points away from the true scores. Therefore, the 3's on the item map are placed at the ability where the expected score is 2.75 and the 0's on the item map are placed at the ability where the expected score is 0.25. These values are thought to represent the useful range of an item. At abilities less than the 0 on the item map the expected score is less than 0.25, indicating that most children of that ability are still scoring 0 on the item and the item is too difficult for children of these abilities. At abilities greater than 3 on the item map the expected score is 2.75, indicating that most children are scoring 3 and the item is easy for children of these abilities.

Figure A6.2 reveals another interesting fact about the relationship between items and expected scores. The location of the expected scores coincides with the location where a score is most likely, for scores of 1 and 2. This is true of all symmetric distributions. The item map can tell you *at what ability* a child is likely to achieve a score, but not *how likely* that score is. In other words, we know that the peak of the probability curve for a score of 1 is located at the expected score of 1, but no information is available about how high that peak is.

The key difference between Thurstone thresholds and expected scores is *how* they describe the difficulty of items. The Thurstone thresholds (and other likelihood thresholds) tell you *how likely* a child of given ability is to succeed on an item. The expected scores tell you *on average* what you can expect a child to achieve.

APPENDIX 7
DISPLAY OF ITEM DIFFICULTIES USING THURSTONE THRESHOLDS

The two figures in this appendix illustrate likelihood thresholds for the items of the GMFM-66. As the name suggests, these figures tell us *how likely* a child with a given ability is to achieve a certain score on a GMFM-66 item. On these plots only the horizontal placement of the items is of importance. There is no *y* axis (ordinate). Rather, for convenience items have been grouped into their GMFM dimensions. Items are stacked on top of each other within a dimension only for ease of illustration. Figure A7.1 shows the Thurstone thresholds for all scores and all items in the GMFM-66. The Thurstone thresholds are the 50% likelihood thresholds. Thus, Figure A7.1 illustrates the ability required to have a 50% chance of achieving each of the item scores in the measure. Figure A7.2 shows the Thurstone thresholds and the 90% likelihood thresholds for scores of 3 only. This figure enables us to see the relative difficulty of completing the items of the GMFM-66.

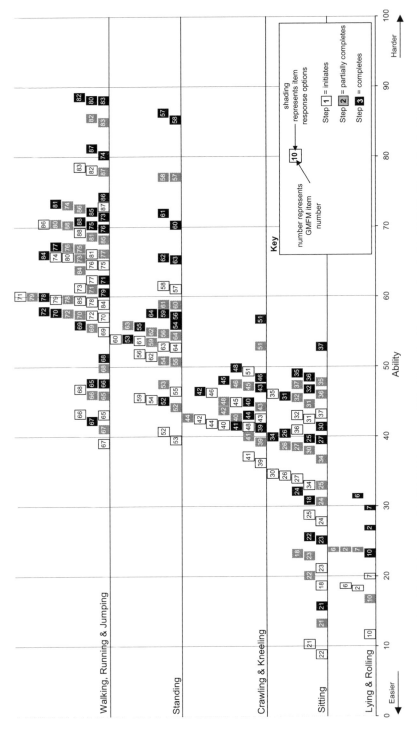

Fig. A7.1. Schematic of GMFM-66 item step difficulties using Thurstone thresholds (50% likelihood thresholds).

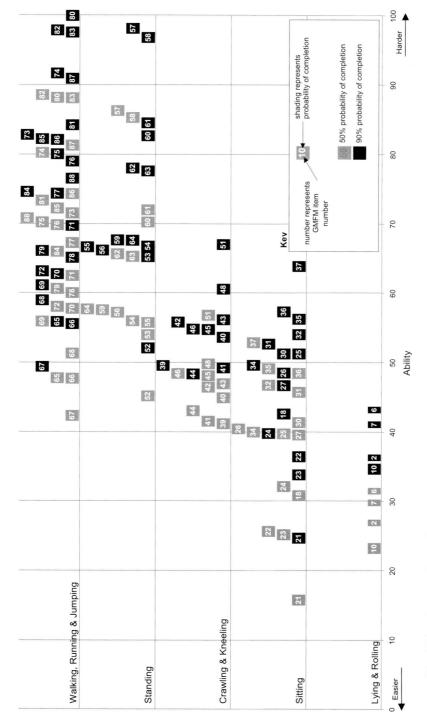

Fig. A7.2. Schematic of the difficulty of completing the items (scoring a 3) on the GMFM-66, using likelihood thresholds of 50% and 90%.

APPENDIX 8
CASE SCENARIO OF TREVOR

Trevor was aged 4.5 years when assessed at the local children's treatment centre in March 1997 prior to starting kindergarten. He has ataxic cerebral palsy but is quite mobile and is classified at level 1 on the GMFCS. As the therapist had never seen Trevor before, she decided to do the 88-item GMFM to get a comprehensive picture of Trevor's gross motor skills.

Trevor scored 100% in the first three dimensions (Lying & Rolling; Sitting, Crawling & Kneeling), and other than some difficulty standing on one foot for more than 3 seconds and getting to standing through half-kneel on his left side he accomplished all the items in the Standing dimension. Trevor can walk up and down steps with the same foot leading consistently and holding the railing but not without holding on. He has difficulty jumping and hopping on one foot. His total GMFM-88 score was 91%.

In September Trevor was reassessed with the GMFM-88. He continued to score 100% on the first three dimensions. His score in the Standing dimension improved by 3%, in the Walking, Running & Jumping dimension by 15%, and his total score by 4%. Trevor was beginning to be able to stand on one foot for several seconds, walk upstairs without using the railing, and jump from a 15cm step without falling.

The information from the GMFM assessments was entered into the GMAE program and the results are summarized in Figures A8.1 to A8.5. Figure A8.5 is the display of the case summary report. At his initial assessment Trevor had a GMFM-66 score of 70.04; at his follow-up assessment he scored 77.46, for a change score of 7.42. The 95% confidence intervals (95% CI) of the March assessment (67.04–73.04) do not overlap with the confidence intervals of the September assessment (73.42–81.5), so we can be fairly confident that the change in Trevor's GMFM-66 score is reflective of true change in his gross motor skills over and above what might be expected from measurement variability.

Figure A8.1 shows the item map by difficulty order of Trevor's initial assessment. His GMFM-66 score of 70 is indicated with a solid vertical line and the 95% CIs are indicated by dashed lines on either side of the solid line. Trevor's item scores are circled in red on the item difficulty map. Looking at the easier items on the GMFM-66 (those mapped at the bottom left hand corner) and following up the difficulty map we can see that Trevor consistently scored 3's until item 61 where he scored a 2. Moving up the map, as the items become more difficult there is some variability of item scores around the vertical line but no scores that are unexpected, with the exception of item 84 (Stand, holding one rail: Walks up four steps, holding one rail, alternating feet) where he scored a 1, whereas based on his total score we might have expected he would score a 2 or 3. We can see that Trevor is scoring 0's on the four most difficult items (hopping on one foot, and using the stairs without holding on to the railing), followed by some 1's and a 2 on the jumping items, which should be the next skills that Trevor is likely to accomplish.

Figure A8.2 shows the item map by item order. It is quickly evident that Trevor accomplishes all items from the Lying & Rolling, Sitting and Crawling & Kneeling dimensions that are part of the GMFM-66. We can see this because all of the easier items have scores of 3 circled. If Trevor had difficulty with an item on the GMFM-88 that was not one of the GMFM-66 items (*e.g.* item 16: Prone: Pivots to right 90° using extremities) it would not be reflected in his GMFM-66 score. When looking at the items in the Standing and Walking, Running & Jumping dimensions we see variability in the scores and know that these are the areas where we might expect Trevor's goals to be focused.

Figures A8.3 and A8.4 are the item maps for Trevor's follow-up assessment. The GMFM-66 score of 77.46 is plotted on both figures with the 95% CIs indicated by the dotted lines on either side of the line. Again, if one scans the scores we get a clear picture of what skills Trevor has accomplished, where there is variability in scores, and what are the gross motor skills Trevor is likely to develop next. There are no unexpected scores.

The data from Trevor's initial and follow-up assessments using the GMFM-66 are summarized in Figure A8.5.

Trevor's GMFM scores and change scores over six months illustrate that, even by assessing only the higher-level items of the GMFM-66, it would be easily possible to obtain an accurate estimate of his progress in gross motor function. In Trevor's case the change in GMFM-66 score (7.42) was greater than the change in his GMFM-88 score (3.5).

Item Map by Difficulty Order

Client ID: 2036
Name: T G
Assessment Date: 07 March 1997
Date of Birth: 08 August 1992
Age: 4y 6m

Gross Motor Function Measure
GMFM-66

GMFM-66 Score: 70.04
Standard Error: 1.53
95% Confidence Interval: 67.04 to 73.04

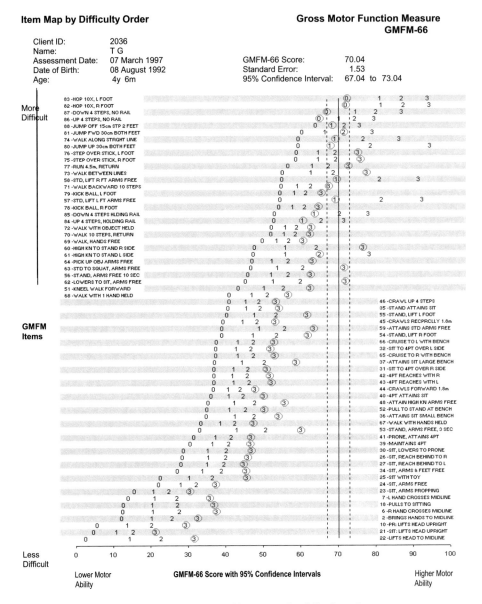

Fig. A8.1. Initial GMFM-66 item map by difficulty order.

220

Item Map by Item Order

Gross Motor Function Measure
GMFM-66

Client ID:	2036
Name:	T G
Assessment Date:	07 March 1997
Date of Birth:	08 August 1992
Age:	4y 6m

GMFM-66 Score:	70.04
Standard Error:	1.53
95% Confidence Interval:	67.04 to 73.04

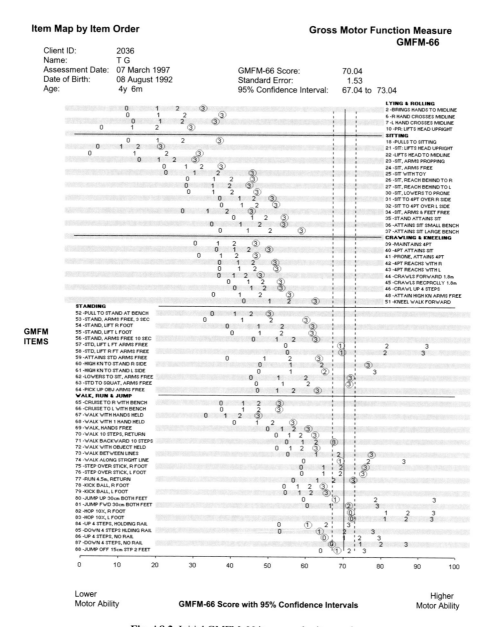

Fig. A8.2. Initial GMFM-66 item map by item order.

221

Item Map by Difficulty Order

Gross Motor Function Measure
GMFM-66

Client ID: 2036
Name: T G
Assessment Date: 09 September 1997
Date of Birth: 08 August 1992
Age: 5y 1m

GMFM-66 Score: 77.46
Standard Error: 2.06
95% Confidence Interval: 73.42 to 81.50

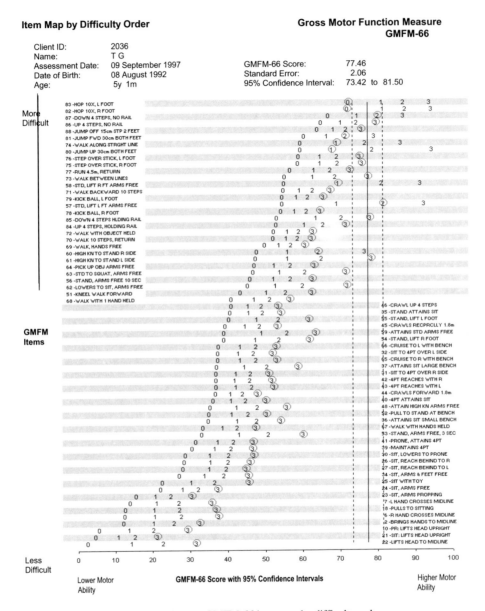

Fig. A8.3. Follow-up GMFM-66 item map by difficulty order.

Item Map by Item Order

Gross Motor Function Measure
GMFM-66

Client ID:	2036
Name:	T G
Assessment Date:	09 September 1997
Date of Birth:	08 August 1992
Age:	5y 1m

GMFM-66 Score:	77.46
Standard Error:	2.06
95% Confidence Interval:	73.42 to 81.50

GMFM ITEMS

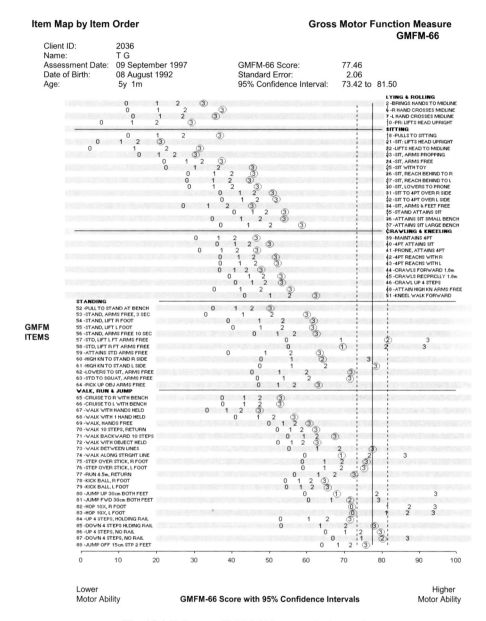

Lower Motor Ability

GMFM-66 Score with 95% Confidence Intervals

Higher Motor Ability

Fig. A8.4. Follow-up GMFM-66 item map by item order.

Case Summary Report

**Gross Motor Function Measure
GMFM-66**

Client ID: 2036
Name: T G
Date of Birth: 08 August 1992
Gender: male
Diagnosis: ataxic

Assessment Date	Age	GMFM-66 Score	Standard Error	95% Confidence Intervals Lower	95% Confidence Intervals Upper	Items Tested	GMFCS	Therapist	Change Score
09 Sep 1997	5y 1m	77.46	2.06	73.42	81.50	66	Level I	NG	7.42
07 Mar 1997	4y 6m	70.04	1.53	67.04	73.04	66	Level I	NC	N/A

Case Summary Plot:

Fig. A8.5. Case summary report.

APPENDIX 9
CASE SCENARIOS OF TWO CHILDREN WHO MISFIT THE GMFM-66 ITEM DIFFICULTY MODEL

The GMFM-66 item maps have been developed by looking at GMFM scores and patterns of GMFM scores from a large number of children with cerebral palsy of varying ages, diagnostic types and severities of motor disability. The item difficulty estimates that are now fixed on the item maps represent the best estimate for the majority of children. It is possible that some children will not fit the model of item difficulty as well as others. The following case scenarios are examples of children who have score distributions that do not follow the pattern that might be expected. It is recommended that you look carefully at the item maps of each child to interpret scores and identify responses that are more variable. There is likely to be a good clinical explanation; however, it is important to note that the child's estimated GMFM-66 score is still the best estimate of their ability.

Clinical scenario 1: Charlie
Charlie is a boy with spastic right hemiparetic cerebral palsy, classified on the GMFCS at level I. He was assessed with the GMFM-66 at age 3 years 9 months, and the findings are displayed in the item maps in Figures A9.1 and A9.2. From these item maps it becomes clear how his gross motor performance could produce the designation as someone who "misfits" the patterns typical of children with cerebral palsy. With a GMFM-66 score of 55, this boy can accomplish a variety of activities. On inspection, however, there are apparent discrepancies between "higher" level skills he does achieve (*e.g.* item 61: "High Kneel: Attains stand through half kneel on left knee, without using arms", or item 77: "Stand: Runs 4.5 m (15 ft), stops and returns") and "lower" level items he is unable to achieve (*e.g.* item 23: "Sit on mat, arm(s) propping: Maintains, 5 seconds", or item 48, "Sit on mat: Attains high kneel using arms, maintains, arms free, 10 seconds").

What will be obvious to people familiar with children with cerebral palsy is that these "gaps" in Charlie's gross motor function are consistent with the impaired function of his right arm and leg. This imposes limitations on him in some aspects of function that ordinarily would be accomplished by a child with a GMFM-66 score of 55, while at the same time not preventing him from accomplishing tasks such as running (item 75) or going down 4 steps holding a rail (item 85). In other words the total GMFM-66 score of 55 is made up of what seems to be a discrepant group of skills and difficulties that are not typical of the majority of children with cerebral palsy whose GMFM data have been used to create these item maps. The clinical scenario associated with the (right) hemisyndrome helps to interpret and "explain" these observations.

Item Map by Difficulty Order

Gross Motor Function Measure
GMFM-66

Client ID: 12020
Name: Charlie
Assessment Date: 21 November 1997
Date of Birth: 12 February 1994
Age: 3y 9m

GMFM-66 Score: 55.15
Standard Error: 1.23
95% Confidence Interval: 52.74 to 57.56

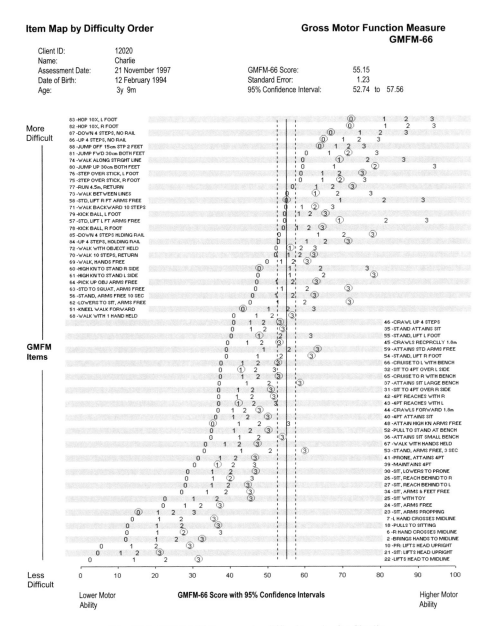

Fig. A9.1. GMFM-66 item map by difficulty order for Charlie.

226

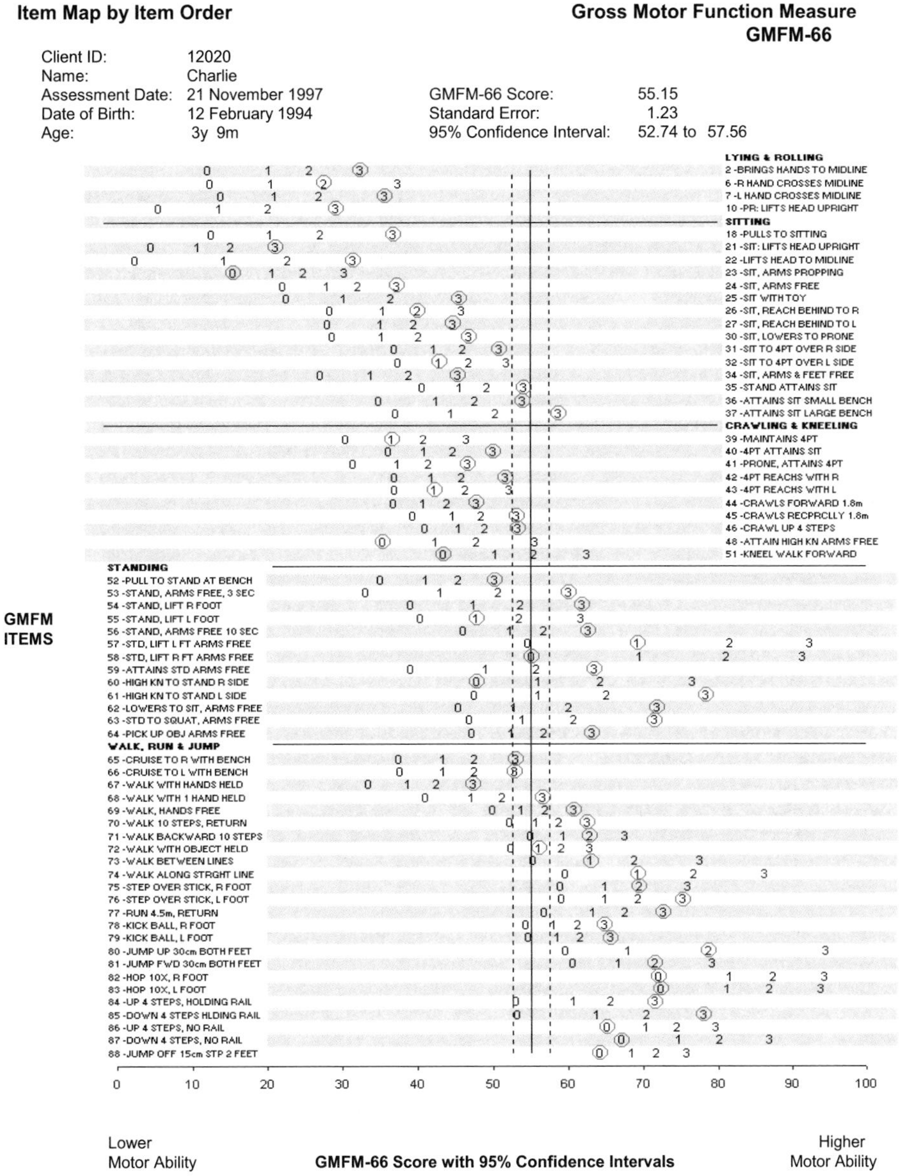

Item Map by Item Order

Gross Motor Function Measure
GMFM-66

Client ID: 12020
Name: Charlie
Assessment Date: 21 November 1997
Date of Birth: 12 February 1994
Age: 3y 9m

GMFM-66 Score: 55.15
Standard Error: 1.23
95% Confidence Interval: 52.74 to 57.56

GMFM ITEMS

LYING & ROLLING
2 -BRINGS HANDS TO MIDLINE
6 -R HAND CROSSES MIDLINE
7 -L HAND CROSSES MIDLINE
10 -PR: LIFTS HEAD UPRIGHT

SITTING
18 -PULLS TO SITTING
21 -SIT: LIFTS HEAD UPRIGHT
22 -LIFTS HEAD TO MIDLINE
23 -SIT, ARMS PROPPING
24 -SIT, ARMS FREE
25 -SIT WITH TOY
26 -SIT, REACH BEHIND TO R
27 -SIT, REACH BEHIND TO L
30 -SIT, LOWERS TO PRONE
31 -SIT TO 4PT OVER R SIDE
32 -SIT TO 4PT OVER L SIDE
34 -SIT, ARMS & FEET FREE
35 -STAND ATTAINS SIT
36 -ATTAINS SIT SMALL BENCH
37 -ATTAINS SIT LARGE BENCH

CRAWLING & KNEELING
39 -MAINTAINS 4PT
40 -4PT ATTAINS SIT
41 -PRONE, ATTAINS 4PT
42 -4PT REACHS WITH R
43 -4PT REACHS WITH L
44 -CRAWLS FORWARD 1.8m
45 -CRAWLS RECPRCLLY 1.8m
46 -CRAWL UP 4 STEPS
48 -ATTAIN HIGH KN ARMS FREE
51 -KNEEL WALK FORWARD

STANDING
52 -PULL TO STAND AT BENCH
53 -STAND, ARMS FREE, 3 SEC
54 -STAND, LIFT R FOOT
55 -STAND, LIFT L FOOT
56 -STAND, ARMS FREE 10 SEC
57 -STD, LIFT L FT ARMS FREE
58 -STD, LIFT R FT ARMS FREE
59 -ATTAINS STD ARMS FREE
60 -HIGH KN TO STAND R SIDE
61 -HIGH KN TO STAND L SIDE
62 -LOWERS TO SIT, ARMS FREE
63 -STD TO SQUAT, ARMS FREE
64 -PICK UP OBJ ARMS FREE

WALK, RUN & JUMP
65 -CRUISE TO R WITH BENCH
66 -CRUISE TO L WITH BENCH
67 -WALK WITH HANDS HELD
68 -WALK WITH 1 HAND HELD
69 -WALK, HANDS FREE
70 -WALK 10 STEPS, RETURN
71 -WALK BACKWARD 10 STEPS
72 -WALK WITH OBJECT HELD
73 -WALK BETWEEN LINES
74 -WALK ALONG STRGHT LINE
75 -STEP OVER STICK, R FOOT
76 -STEP OVER STICK, L FOOT
77 -RUN 4.5m, RETURN
78 -KICK BALL, R FOOT
79 -KICK BALL, L FOOT
80 -JUMP UP 30cm BOTH FEET
81 -JUMP FWD 30cm BOTH FEET
82 -HOP 10X, R FOOT
83 -HOP 10X, L FOOT
84 -UP 4 STEPS, HOLDING RAIL
85 -DOWN 4 STEPS HLDING RAIL
86 -UP 4 STEPS, NO RAIL
87 -DOWN 4 STEPS, NO RAIL
88 -JUMP OFF 15cm STP 2 FEET

0   10   20   30   40   50   60   70   80   90   100

Lower
Motor Ability

GMFM-66 Score with 95% Confidence Intervals

Higher
Motor Ability

Fig. A9.2. GMFM-66 item map by item order for Charlie.

227

Case scenario 2: Sarah

Sarah has cerebral palsy, described as spastic diplegia. She was determined to be functioning at level III on the GMFCS. Sarah was assessed on her sixth birthday, and the item maps reflecting her skills and limitations are shown in Figures A9.3 and A9.4. There is a striking pattern of accomplishments and apparent failures to do activities well below the observed GMFM-66 score of almost 47. These can be seen most clearly on the item map by item order, where it is evident that Sarah is unable to accomplish any of the Crawling & Kneeling items, although she scores 3's on a number of items that involve standing and on a few walking items. It is therefore not surprising to learn that, in addition to her seizure disorder and overall developmental slowness, Sarah has significant visual functional difficulties that almost certainly contribute to her floor-level functional limitations. In walking she might be able to use her hands for guidance, whereas in floor-level mobility this would be extremely difficult and would make it very likely that she would remain immobile on the floor. It is for this reason that she would be classified as a child who "misfits" the data.

Item Map by Difficulty Order

Gross Motor Function Measure
GMFM-66

Client ID: 13043
Name: Sarah
Assessment Date: 08 October 1996
Date of Birth: 07 October 1990
Age: 6y 0m

GMFM-66 Score: 46.91
Standard Error: 1.05
95% Confidence Interval: 44.85 to 48.97

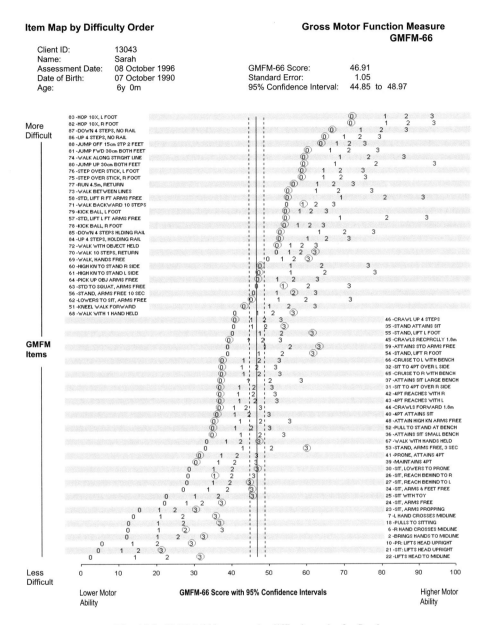

Fig. A9.3. GMFM-66 item map by difficulty order for Sarah.

Item Map by Item Order

Gross Motor Function Measure
GMFM-66

Client ID: 13043
Name: Sarah
Assessment Date: 08 October 1996
Date of Birth: 07 October 1990
Age: 6y 0m

GMFM-66 Score: 46.91
Standard Error: 1.05
95% Confidence Interval: 44.85 to 48.97

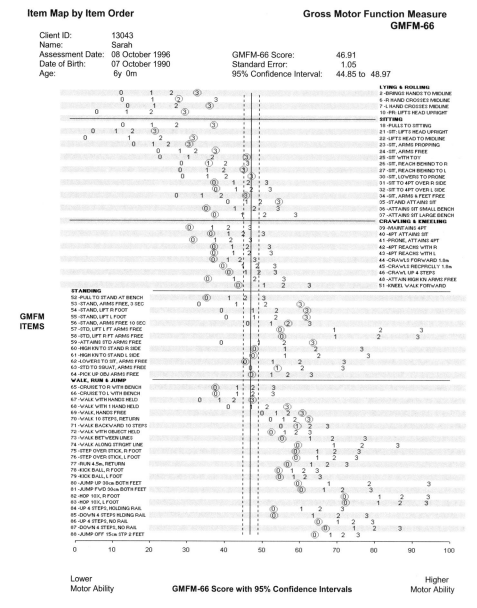

GMFM ITEMS

Lower
Motor Ability

GMFM-66 Score with 95% Confidence Intervals

Higher
Motor Ability

Fig. A9.4. GMFM-66 item map by item order for Sarah.

230

INDEX

(Page numbers in *italics* refer to figures/tables.)

233